Jenni Murray has been a regular presenter of Radio 4's *Woman's Hour* since 1987. She also presents *Weekend Woman's Hour* each Saturday. In the Queen's Birthday Honours 1999 she was awarded an OBE for radio broadcasting.

Jenni is the author of *The Woman's Hour*, a history of women since World War II. She contributes to numerous newspapers and magazines and is an occasional documentary film-maker.

D0064557

Is it me,
or is it hot in here?

A modern woman's guide
to the menopause

Jenni Murray

Vermilion
LONDON

DEDICATION

I dedicate this book to my agent, Barbara Levy, who is a prop beyond the call of duty and for whom the book has become a bible, and to Liz Senior, my indefatiguable researcher who is only 26 but will one day be the best informed perimenopausal woman in the world (and it will come, Liz. I promise, one day, you too will be able to say 'Is it me?' and I will groan 'No, it's bloody hot in here').

7 9 10 8 6

Text copyright © Jenni Murray 2001

The right of Jenni Murray to be identified as the author of this book has been asserted by her in accordance with the Copyright, Designs and Patent Act 1988.

First published in the United Kingdom in 2001 by Vermilion
an imprint of Ebury Press
Random House, 20 Vauxhall Bridge Road, London SW1V 2SA
www.randomhouse.co.uk
This edition is published in 2003

Random House Australia (Pty) Limited
20 Alfred Street, Milsons Point, Sydney, New South Wales 2061, Australia

Random House New Zealand Limited
18 Poland Road, Glenfield, Auckland 10, New Zealand

Random House (Pty) Limited
Isle of Houghton, Corner of Boundary Road & Carse O'Gowrie,
Houghton 2198, South Africa

The Random House Group Limited Reg. No. 954009

A CIP catalogue record for this book is available from the British Library
'Menopause' by Jean Earle is taken from *Selected Poems* (Seren, 1990)

ISBN 9780091887773

The Random House Group Limited supports The Forest Stewardship Council (FSC), the leading international forest certification organisation. All our titles that are printed on Greenpeace approved FSC certified paper carry the FSC logo. Our paper procurement policy can be found at:
www.rbooks.co.uk/environment

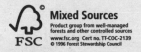

Mixed Sources
Product group from well-managed forests and other controlled sources
www.fsc.org Cert no. TT-COC-2139
© 1996 Forest Stewardship Council

Typeset in Goudy by SX Composing DTP, Rayleigh, Essex
Printed and bound in Great Britain by Cox & Wyman Ltd, Reading, Berkshire

Contents

Introduction   6

Chapter 1: What is the menopause?   9

Chapter 2: How the menopause became a battleground   42

Chapter 3: Trust me, I'm a doctor   75

Chapter 4: What is HRT?   107

Chapter 5: The pros and cons of HRT   142

Chapter 6: The alternatives to HRT   177

Chapter 7: Diet and exercise   216

Chapter 8: Old age ain't for cissies   263

Further Reading   281

Useful Addresses   283

Index   286

INTRODUCTION

'Is it me or is it hot in here?' Words I first uttered, in genuine discomfort, during an extremely hot, outside summer broadcast, only a couple of years ago. The grin of recognition which broke out around the hall was warming – which was a pity given the circumstances. The grin turned into full-bellied laughter from the studio audience and resulted in 3000 sympathetic letters from people listening at home, thanking me for being brave enough to mention a hot flush in such a public arena.

I have to say, I hadn't realised until then that the menopause was still such a taboo, to be moaned about in private with one's best mates, but never shouted from the roof tops. (You are no doubt reading this, covered in brown paper with an inky title, perhaps *Latin Primer for First Formers*. A sort of latter-day *Lady Chatterley*, to be passed, unobserved, around your girlfriends!)

But, didn't Mrs Thatcher run the country, allegedly keeping the HRT industry extremely buoyant during her tour of duty? She was praised, even by her arch-political enemy, Shirley Williams, for the model she set for women of a certain age.

When I look back and think of when women as possible Prime Ministers were first discussed, I remember that one of the arguments always made was that they would probably come to power at the time when women have the menopause and they would be incapable of making any decisions. Mrs Thatcher, presumably, at one stage or another went through the menopause. There was not a single indication that she did and one never saw anything in her behaviour that would suggest the slightest ups and downs. Since then, no one has ever said women can't be tough enough to be politicians.

The letters suggested, though, that Thatcher, the glowing Teresa Gorman, the heavenly Helen Mirren gracing the front page of *Radio Times* in her birthday suit, proclaiming she was Fabulous and Fifty, or Germaine Greer claiming the right to become a crone, were not enough to convince the rest of us that the Change was something to be spoken of in polite society.

There's a hidden fear, I suspect, that if we're open about it, someone will question our right to be out there, fresh-faced and full of ourselves, on top of the job, planning a climb up Everest or rowing across the Atlantic and they'll send us back where we belong – wearing black in a darkened room, greying, knitting, sliding into cantankerous, brittle-boned senility.

But we are the Baby Boomers, the ones who rode on the coat-tails of second wave feminism and reaped the benefits of the radical seeds they sowed. They tried out the pill, opened up the workplace, threw their stilettos in the bin (although I'm told no one ever actually burned a bra), made childbirth a potentially humane experience where we wrestled back some control and test-drove HRT.

Thus, when I became perimenopausal – the one to two years when you start to feel a bit down and the periods can become erratic and heavy, but don't stop – I knew to trot along to the doctor's and make enquiries. A blood test later, I was told, 'Yes, you're clearly menopausal. What do you want, pills or patches?' And thanks to the sisters with challenging minds who'd gone before, I knew not to accept the medicalisation of my 'problem' as a given. I took pills for a bit, tried patches for a while and I'm having a go with natural progesterone. The medication helped the depression, but the hot flushes and night sweats are still humungous – and that's nearly five years on. I still can't pass a mirror and see my grandmother – thickened waist, specs and slightly sagging chin – and quite believe it's me.

Now it's a question of checking on the bones with a density test and organising a diet and exercise that will sustain the energy levels, keep me out of the orthopaedic ward and maybe reduce my weight again. I still can't decide whether or not to go back on HRT.

As in every other area of life for women of my age, there are choices. Given today's longer life spans, lots of us will be post-menopausal for a third of our lives. As we bring up our children so much later we'll have to deal with that explosive hormonal cocktail, the menopausal woman and the teenage son or daughter. We'll have to decide whether we want to go along with science that seeks to keep us young and nubile, either through pills and potions or the surgeon's knife, whether we want to grow old disgracefully with a hairdresser with a great line in hair dye as our constant companion, or whether we'll be graceful and grey in the distinguished manner so far only open to the male of the species.

We'll discuss all these options in this menopause manual – and just remember one thing if you begin to waver and wonder whether the post-menopausal period will be worth living – you are never, ever going to have to worry again about getting pregnant. No more pills, caps, agonising over terminations or fiddling with condoms (unless you're really planning a high old time). Women's Liberation proper begins here.

CHAPTER 1

WHAT IS THE
MENOPAUSE?

In the late 1980s, at the age of 49, one of Britain's best-known and best respected actors, an award-winning international star of stage and screen and now a busy Member of Parliament, missed a period. 'Jesus Christ' – her heart flipped over in horror – 'I must be pregnant.' A moment of calm consideration convinced her that this couldn't possibly be the case. Immaculate conception was, she conceded, unlikely. 'So, that's it,' she told herself, 'the menopause.'

In Glenda Jackson's case it was, indeed, the menopause, although if this happens to you, and you are sexually active, it is worth having a pregnancy test just to be sure – even if you are past the age when you thought you might still be fertile. Of every 20 women between the ages of 40 and 55 seen in a doctor's surgery complaining of missed or irregular periods, 19 of them will not be pregnant. Which means, of course, that one of them will be. One GP, by the way, recently told me how astonished she is at the number of women, even in the 21st century, who come to her surgery in a complete tizzy, complaining of heavier, more irregular periods, or of their sudden absence. They wonder what on earth is wrong with them and menopause, she says, often never crosses their minds. Which is what this book is all about: information and shared experience, so that you know what's happening to you and can make choices about what action to take.

Generally, you would not be expected to be sterile, unless you've undergone an operation for that purpose or have had a hysterectomy, until you have been menstruation-free for a year over the age of 50, or two years under 50. Younger women with typical symptoms might believe themselves safe, but it's not unknown for them to begin having periods again after what they thought might be menopause. So it's as well to continue with contraception until you're certain that you are post-menopausal. Your doctor can usually confirm this by taking a blood test to establish the levels of the follicle-stimulating hormone (FSH), which tend be higher after the menopause, but lower in women whose periods may have stopped temporarily due to severe weight loss or stress.

If you suspect you may be pregnant, be a little wary of some over-the-counter pregnancy tests which can, in older age groups, give false positives. Don't panic. Go to a doctor you trust. Equally, abnormal pregnancies such as ectopics can give false negatives with some types of test. Again – be safe, not sorry, and see a doctor in good time if you think you may be pregnant. Leaving it too late will preclude the possibility of carrying out certain genetic investigations to check the health of the foetus. It may also rule out early termination, which you may want to consider if you can't face starting again with a new baby in your forties or even early fifties. If in doubt, check it out.

As Glenda pondered the preceding weeks and months, she realised that her periods, although regular, had been quite heavy for a while and there had been a few nights when, as she puts it, she had woken up wrapped in 'sodden sheets', but she really hadn't paid it too much attention. In fact, she had barely thought about it at all. Now she felt an immense sense of relief that she wouldn't have to bother with 'all that' any more, chucked out the sanitary products that littered her bathroom and 'got on with life'.

Glenda rightly identifies the meaning of the word 'menopause'. It derives from the Greek *meno*, meaning month, and pausis, which means ending. It refers to one date, the last day of your final period, and can consequently only be pinned down retrospectively. Menopause is generally assumed to have been completed when a clear year has passed, period-free. As the writer Germaine Greer describes it: 'The word menopause applies to a non-event, the menstrual period that does not happen.'

Few of us, I suspect, will ever have taken the trouble, as we often failed to when we were trying to have children, to mark down the day exactly – with the result that the precise timing of the menopause becomes as vague for most of us as was the due delivery date for our kids. So, if you really want to know for future reference, start jotting down in your diary – now.

It would have come in handy in my case. I'm taking part in a trial of natural progesterone (more later), primarily because of my interest in alternative therapies, but mainly for a thorough MOT (mammogram, endometrial aspiration – the worst test known to woman, involving removal of a tiny bit of the lining of the womb via the cervix without anaesthetic. Yuk! Ouch! – pelvic ultrasound scan, which can reveal ovarian cancer, blood tests, blood pressure monitoring, etc). Any clinical trial has to make sure you're fully healthy before using you as a human guinea pig. It makes you sound really dim when they ask, 'And when was the date of your last period?' and you have to make it up. 'Sort of Aprilish, last year,' was the best I could do. I think they were used to hearing it, but it does help if you can be precise about it.

It is perhaps a little premature to toss out the tampons after the first missed period. It's quite common, indeed it happened to me, to go for a whole year and then find your body has just one final fling – fooled you! – and you have to count all over again for another year to be considered, officially, a post-menopausal woman. Christine Clancy, the tea-pourer on the September page of the Rylstone WI calendar, tells me her periods stopped suddenly when she was 46 with absolutely no prior warning. She was free for a year and then the rogue one, almost a year to the day, came right at the beginning of a week's holiday with her husband John in Majorca. They have no children, so were looking forward to a romantic fling. It was not to be and, of course, she was taken totally by surprise. Best, as every good Girl Guide knows, to Be Prepared!

There are other terms which are often used to identify this time in a woman's life. 'The Change' was the favoured designation of my childhood, muttered conspiratorially by middle-aged aunts who mopped the beads of sweat from their brows with freshly laundered and starched, lace-edged handkerchiefs and, unnaturally pink of cheek, complained of the heat in the days long before central heating. Vera Ivers OBE, chair of the steering committee for the Older Women's Network UK (OWN), remembers her mother and aunts gossiping in condemnatory whispers about one of their number, 'Why does she keep going on long shopping trips when she keeps flooding?' 'She's going through the Change, you know.'

It would never have occurred to a girl to ask what they were talking about, although the tone said it all. A change for the worse. Dangerous, depressing, a descent into useless tittle-tattle over tea and scones, bemoaning the waywardness of absent adult children and the woes of caring for ailing husbands or dying parents. Nothing to look forward to. It's not a word I would choose to use at all.

Although she calls her book on the subject, *The Change*, Germaine Greer favours a terminology which, like menopause, derives from the Greek. 'Climacteric' is rooted in klimacter, meaning critical period, and refers to the ten years, usually from 45 to 55, when the majority of us make our transition from reproductive to non-reproductive creatures. For me it still accentuates the negative, rather than the positive. 'Critical' has associations with illness, accidents, descent.

There's nothing in 'climacteric' to reflect a new and welcome tone in depictions of women in middle age which, for the past few years, have begun to be the norm. The American feminist Gloria Steinem started the trend when, in the late 1980s, she published a photograph of herself in the bath in celebration of her birthday and proudly proclaimed, 'This is what 50 looks like.' Helen Mirren stunningly did the same in the 1990s on the front page of the *Radio Times*.

In New Year 2000 came the 'calendar pin-up girls' of the Rylstone WI, unashamedly revealing flesh way past the first flush of youth, but with pride and a wicked sense of humour. In the summer of the same year *Good Housekeeping* magazine referred to women in their forties and fifties not as middle-aged, but as 'grown up'. This was followed by a feature in the *Sunday Express*, accompanied by photographs of the actress Kathleen Turner, who famously stripped off in *The Graduate* on the London stage, Harriet Harman MP and Camilla Parker Bowles, resplendent in pink Versace.

None of these women is conventionally pretty. Turner is quite plump, Camilla has always been a surprisingly Plain Jane choice of sex siren mistress for a Prince of Wales and Harman is the jolly hockey sticks head girl lookalike she's always been. But the article was headlined 'Women's Lib? It Really Starts in Middle Age'. The women were described as older and sexier, difficult to control and independent-minded.

Perhaps 'metamorphosis' would be a more suitable handle for this time of life for us all. A change for the better, leaving behind the confining chrysalis of anxiety about being overburdened double shifters, bound by biology to a constant fear of pregnancy and a monthly cycle that, if we're honest, at best bores us, at worst drives us temporarily barmy with the moon. As the magazine editor Marcelle d'Argy Smith observes, 'Women are like eggs. They hatch in their forties.'

There are, of course, for most of us, some grotty bits to go through before we reach menstruation-free nirvana. When Glenda Jackson talked about the hot sweats and heavy bleeding she experienced, she pinned down two of the common symptoms of the perimenopausal period and – in the case of the hot flushes – sometimes of the post-menopausal period too. (Perimenopause can extend from a few months to several years and refers to the time when we first observe changes to the menstrual cycle. It usually lasts for about a year after the last period.)

Hot flushes, night sweats and palpitations are thought to be experienced by 70 per cent of women for a year, 30 per cent for five years and 5-10 per cent for 10 years. After an induced menopause, where the ovaries are surgically removed, almost all women will have severe hot flushes, beginning immediately after surgery, regardless of their age. In a natural menopause, flushes usually begin in the late forties, but can start earlier and can go on for as little as a year or as long as 15 years – although that's rare, you'll be relieved to know. Like adolescence, where the body and the mind set are adjusting to a new reproductive role, the 'metamorphosis' can take several years, during which we can learn to accommodate ourselves as a new and different kind of woman with time and energy to follow our own inclinations rather than those of the people who have depended upon us in the past.

Hot flushes generally have a consistent pattern, but manifest themselves differently in each individual woman. They can last for two to three minutes or up to an hour and can come several times a day or only occasionally (mine come at night, or at a party or an important business meeting. I find a joky 'Is it me or is it hot in here?', a sweet smile, and a tissue to mop the fevered brow, invaluable and much less embarrassing than trying to conceal what's going on! Lightweight clothing is essential. Don't bother with expensive silk shirts, you'll only ruin them, and I have drawers full of sweaters that I'm looking forward to wearing some time in the future when this inbuilt central heating runs out of fuel and hypothermia sets in! I just hope they'll still fit, but that's another story!)

Glenda Jackson was lucky and, from my conversations with a great range of women, relatively rare, in that her symptoms were quite mild and continued for a short time. Her fellow MP from the other side of the house, Teresa Gorman, says her first indication came in her mid to late forties, when her memory became very poor. She's a scientist and knowing the generic names for the plants in her garden was second nature to her. Suddenly she couldn't tell her *Cistus creticus* from her *Nicotiana sylvestris*. She was running her own business and was used to being interested in everything; indeed she was known for her phenomenal energy, sense of humour and bright outlook. For the first time in her life, her desk was piling up with things to do and she wasn't getting on with them. She was sneaking off to bed, exhausted, at 7 o'clock in the evening, interested in nothing but going to sleep.

She also suffered inklings of hot flushes but, more worryingly, pains in her joints, which she thought might be the early onset of arthritis or rheumatism. She had difficulty climbing the 75 steps in her London town house thanks to stiffness in her knees and hips, and her wrists, in particular, became a problem. She avoided using knives because cutting, chopping and peeling became so painful (sounds like an excuse to bunk off the cooking to me. I had similar problems, and used them to good effect! Luckily, him indoors is a great cook too.)

Moyra Livesey – Miss May, the flower-arranger, in the WI calendar – reports a similar deterioration in her memory and mental processes. She says she couldn't think of words of more than two syllables and became afraid to take an active part in meetings any more as she found herself stuck for simple means of expression. She remembers one particular gathering of the WI where she couldn't remember the name of a very close friend and had to nudge a neighbour to ask the 'dark-haired woman in the green sweater' to turn around and speak to her. Her night sweats were horrendous and her poor husband would shiver on freezing cold nights as she tossed off the bedclothes. It was, she says, as if someone had turned the heating up full-blast. She went off sex completely, mainly because she couldn't stand the heat of her husband's body, but regained the physical side of her relationship post-menopausally.

Only one person I have spoken to has suffered from the vaginal dryness that is reported as a symptom in most of the books I've read, and even in her case the symptom disappeared of its own accord after the menopause. The latest research suggests that it can be a factor for some women, as oestrogen deficiency (the attributed cause of the menopause) is said to be influential in a number of urogenital problems. It's said, in some cases, to result in thinner and paler mucus which can cause itching and what are charmingly described as pelvic laxity and stress incontinence. Is it my naturally suspicious mind that leads me to suspect that it's extremely useful for the marketing department at KY Jelly for this to be promulgated as common? Especially when most of us know that a few pelvic floor exercises (for laxity or incontinence) or letting the imagination substitute George Clooney for the old man (for any dryness that might be a problem) can work miracles! I often find that books on the subject either don't include women's personal experience or are written by men. I guess it wouldn't occur to them to look to their own laurels in this department.

Melba Wilson, who at the age of 50 became policy director for the mental health charity, MIND, had the classic hot flushes and night sweats, but says that in her case her menopausal changes largely involved her sexuality. She's been married to Jake for 25 years and they have had a happy, energetic and physically satisfying relationship throughout. Suddenly she found she wasn't interested at all. Primarily, it was her reduced energy levels – she was so focused on the intricacies of her new job, she could only see bed as a place to slumber. She also became very tired because the night sweats caused her sleep to be disturbed. Few of us would feel like an energetic sex life if we were simply exhausted.

Jake was very upset at her seeming lack of interest in him. Nevertheless, she found she couldn't react the way she had when, earlier in their marriage, after her pregnancies, she had also gone off the physical side of her relationship. As a younger woman she had felt apologetic and ploughed ahead, even though she wasn't necessarily enthusiastic. Now she found herself being more assertive and just saying no. It is, she says, good to have arrived at a point where she is demanding more for herself and is convinced the physical unpleasantness of menopausal symptoms have a purpose in contributing to a woman becoming less accommodating, more demanding and more sure of herself.

There was also an up side to her partial abstinence. When they did get it together, it was better than ever, with hitherto undreamed-of multiple orgasms (she doesn't know why). It is, she insists, important to articulate all these thoughts and feelings with partners, otherwise they can feel extremely lost and left out, which is when the temptation comes for men to diminish or dismiss the powerful transformation that is taking place in the woman's body and mind with a joke. Or, in the worst possible case, decide they'll seek their comfort elsewhere!

Vera Ivers was in the first years of a new second marriage to a man 12 years her junior when her menopause began and reports no difficulties in her sex life. Now she's 68 and it still hasn't come to an end. There are, she says, days when they don't bother at all, but when it happens it's comforting and comfortable. Vera had a hysterectomy in her late thirties after the very difficult birth of her fourth child. A growth was discovered, so she happily went along with the recommendation that she should have her womb removed. Obviously her periods finished as a result of the hysterectomy, so when she got the other classic menopausal symptoms such as flushes and night sweats at the age of 50 it was a bit of a shock, even though her gynaecologist had, she now recalls, told her at the time of the operation that they would leave her ovaries behind, as they were not diseased, and this way she 'would not age suddenly'. She does emphasise out that hysterectomy should never be thought of as making you less of a woman. As she says, it's the clitoris and vagina, not the uterus or the cervix that play a part in sexual stimulation, and orgasm and libido originate from the central nervous system. So whether you fancy someone is in your head, not your womb!

Rosie Thomas is a best-selling novelist whose husband of 30 years left her soon after her menopause, but she now has a new boyfriend, with whom she says sex is 'just fine'. It leads me to suspect that, where there are problems of dryness, it's often likely to be boredom or overfamiliarity rather than physical incapacity that causes a lack of response to sexual stimuli. If you're with the same partner you've been with for many years, you're beginning to feel like an unalluring beached whale and it bothers you, talk about it with your partner, as Melba Wilson recommends, as a first line of attack. Leaving it unspoken will only make the problem fester and get worse.

Later in the book we'll discuss ways of making yourself feel better with diet, exercise and hormonal treatments if you want to try them. Of course, some women say they really don't mind slowing down sexually at this time of life and, if they're really honest, neither do their partners. Men, too, are affected by their hormones and their potency and desire can often fade with age. The trick here would seem to be to try and match each other. No point bumping up your hormonal intake if he's happy to read, drink cocoa and grow old gracefully. Not every fella wants to become Viagra-man, just as we don't all want HRT.

Rosie's menopause was, perhaps, the most frightening, and certainly the most dramatic symptomatically, of anyone's in my wide-ranging sample. She was taking part in the Peking to Paris Motor challenge when she developed perimenopausal uterine haemorrhaging. She was 49 and when she began bleeding heavily she put it down to 'that time of life'. As she drove on through the Himalayas the bleeding became worse and at Everest camp she haemorrhaged severely. She was very ill and describes herself feeling scared and a little ethereal.

A phone call to her gynaecologist in London was not encouraging. He told her the probable cause was a severe and uncommon drop in hormone levels and ordered her to get the first flight home. Her 32-year-old male travelling companion was none too impressed either. She, though, is not a woman to be easily deflected from a challenge. In Kathmandu, by an extraordinary stroke of good luck, she found a traveller who happened to be carrying progestogen pills, borrowed some, felt better and knew instinctively that she was going to be all right. She carried on to Paris and completed the contest. On her return home she was fitted with a progestogen coil which was inserted into the uterus and she's been in perfect health ever since. Hers was not, perhaps, a course of action to be recommended to everyone, but it is an indication that this age need be no barrier to an intrepid and determined nature.

Moyra Livesey describes another common experience. She refuses to call it depression but, with typical Yorkshire understatement, will go so far as to say she was 'very down'. Her husband, looking back on that time, recalls her going from nice to nasty in ten seconds flat. Her teenage son who, mercifully, she says, is a fairly calm, laid-back sort of chap, remembers her reaction to his typically untidy bedroom. One day she'd be fine about it, the next she would scream and shout. Similarly, if the house was untidy or the washing up hadn't been done, some days she took it in her stride; other days she couldn't bear it. She was, she says, totally irrational and difficult to live with.

For me, this was the hardest part of my own menopausal symptoms. At the age of 46, with no prior warning and no history of depressive illness, I woke up one morning looking into a black tunnel with no light at the end. Nothing in my life had changed to induce such misery. My job appeared safe and was as enjoyable as ever, my children were hale and hearty, my parents fit and well, my partnership of nearly 20 years was solid and satisfying. Nevertheless, for several months, every wakening was a sock in the stomach and every programme a huge effort of will. The garden ceased to give me pleasure. I couldn't concentrate to read a book. The family avoided me and the poisonous black cloud that hung around me.

One of my closest friends, Griselda Cann, wrote me an e-mail when we were going through this time. It read thus:

> Your brain cannot be as bad as mine. [It always was a competitive friendship!] Menopause for me means thermonuclear breakdown of all my regulators, intermittent but utter loss of vocabulary, shipwrecked sleep, spatial disorientation, jibbering articulation, shakes, collapse of inner self, extremely vivid dreams and imaging during so-called day time, so that I get preoccupied with irrelevant thoughts when I ought to be concentrating on this or that, and a general lack of grip. AAAAAAAGGGGGHHHHH! I should have added in the extraordinary aches and scrapiness of all my muscles and joints. I imagine myself with brain tumour, impending heart attack, certainly Alzheimer's, thrombosis, arthritis, or perhaps it's not imaginary. Oh God.

In the Western world the majority of women will experience 'natural menopause' (one that is not brought about by any form of medical intervention) between the ages of 45 and 55, but on average around the age of 51. Some women reach menopause earlier in their forties and a few last out until their sixties. Menopause is considered premature if it occurs under the age of 40.

Gail Jones, who is now 42 and works with children with special needs, had the earliest symptoms I have come across so far. She married in her early twenties and had her second child at 25. Almost immediately she began to feel 'peculiar'. Like Moyra and me, she's not the sort of person who has ever suffered from depression, but she began to feel very low. She became afraid of driving her car and, in fact, felt tired, anxious and fearful all the time. She was nauseous and had difficulty swallowing. Her hair began to thin, she had headaches and hot flushes, aches in her breasts and intercourse became painful – probably because she was so full of fear. She frequently suffered from cystitis. Her periods became erratic with a shorter than usual space between them and she sometimes experienced flooding. She began to feel, she says, like a completely sexless person, obsessed in the worst possible way with her nether regions. Her symptoms were explained away as post-natal depression, until, two years later, her periods stopped.

Gail had a pregnancy test which proved negative and, after much 'fobbing off' by the NHS, decided to pay for specialist investigations of what she thought might be a life-threatening illness. Eventually, after extensive tests for every known condition, she was told she was menopausal. She then discovered that her sister had also gone through the same process at the age of 32, although their mother had had a normal change at 50.

There was no explanation for such a young woman mirroring the patterns of someone usually twice her age, except that she was told her experience was unquestionably hereditary – that both she and her sister must carry a 'throwback gene'. When she was finally given the diagnosis it was a huge relief. She was disappointed that she wouldn't be able to have more children, but, since her most fervent wish during these two years of hell had been to be spared until she was 40 so that she could bring up the two kids she'd had, she was relieved and delighted to be told her life was not in danger.

It's common to experience symptoms at around the same age as mothers and sisters – so it's a great help if you have them around to talk to. Mothers can be problematic, though. Menopause seems to be rather like childbirth – once it's over you forget about the pain and horrors and concentrate on the challenge of being the new you, so don't be surprised if your mum, like mine, is spectacularly vague about what to you seems the most dramatic time in your life since adolescence and childbirth, as indeed it is.

Apart from genetics, the only consistent factor shown to affect the age at menopause is cigarette-smoking. Smokers (and even ex-smokers) can reach menopause two or three years earlier than those who have never indulged. Contrary to earlier medical opinion, there is no link between the time of a woman's first period and her age at menopause, nor is there any proven connection between the use of oral contraceptives and the onset of symptoms.

Penny Heeley, who's a fitness instructor at the Ragdale Hall Health Hydro in Leicestershire, and whose exercise programme for health in the middle years you can find later in the book (see p. 255), started taking the pill in 1969, at a relatively high dose, came off it for a while in the early 1970s when she had her son, transferred to a low dose in 1974 and continued to take it without a break until she was 52. Her doctor then suggested she might safely come off it without risk of pregnancy, which she did, and she hasn't had a period since. She's now 53 and, apart from one night sweat and one occasion when she had what she describes as a panic attack in a shopping mall where she had to rush out to be able to breathe, she has been symptom-free and is as well balanced and fit as it's possible to be.

The timing of the menopause can often be accelerated by traumatic events. Prolonged stress or a life crisis can halt the production of certain hormones, stop periods temporarily or, in some cases, induce an early menopause. Nutrition can also play an important role. As with the anorexic teenager whose periods stop as she starves herself, an older woman who has been under-nourished for a prolonged period is likely to become menopausal several years earlier than her fellows and anyone who has suffered severe anorexia is at risk of premature menopause.

Leni Pickles, seen repotting her plants on the April page of the WI calendar, began to have symptoms relatively young, at the age of 42. She's a smoker and she thinks both her mother and elder sister had theirs quite early too, although she isn't sure. It's not really something they've talked about much. Most significantly, her husband left her just before she first missed a period. It was a terrible shock. She had three young children: a girl of 16, a boy of 11 and a daughter of 4. She had a full-time job as a lecturer in Social Studies at a nearby college of further education and the first thing she knew about her husband's affair was when he didn't come home one night. He then announced that he had left her for a woman 15 years her junior.

After this her periods became erratic, she felt very tired all the time and began to have the occasional hot flush. Her first thought was that she was coming down with something nasty and then it occurred to her that she might be menopausal. She went to her doctor for a blood test which proved negative. Nine months later, as her periods became increasingly erratic – some long, some short, some missed altogether – she returned for another blood test and was now declared perimenopausal. Looking back, she feels, it's clear that the stress of picking up the pieces of her life as a lone parent may well have been the trigger.

As we've already seen, a hysterectomy usually does not have the effect of precipitating menopause unless the ovaries have been removed. Even when only a portion of ovary is left behind you should expect things to take their normal course. Sandy Chalmers, a former editor of *Woman's Hour*, now Director of

Communications for Help the Aged and Chairman of the Board of Trustees for the Pennell Initiative for Women's Health, began to suffer from debilitating periods in her mid forties. She became tired and anaemic. A D & C (dilation and curettage) proved ineffective, so a hysterectomy was recommended. She was in such a tizzy, she didn't discuss what would happen with her surgeon before the operation, but remembers being told afterwards that half an ovary had been left behind in order that she would have a natural menopause, saving the need for hormone replacement therapy in a relatively young woman.

Of around 90,000 hysterectomies carried out in Britain each year, oopherectomy, or removal of the ovaries, takes place in some 14 per cent of cases, even when they are healthy and free of disease. It is more common if the woman is in her fifties and post menopausal, although it has also occurred in some high-profile and highly controversial cases involving younger women. Some surgeons will suggest there are benefits to oophorectomy. Ovarian cancer is notoriously difficult to diagnose in its early stages, so some doctors will argue that, whilst they are in there, they may as well remove the ovaries and rule out the possibility of any future malignancy, or of ovarian cysts developing. Other doctors will be happier to leave healthy ovaries in place, to prevent the symptoms of menopause arriving before their time, although this is not guaranteed. The most recent data show that 50 per cent of ovaries fail to function after hysterectomy.

Informed consent has proved to be a key problem here. Some women have thought they were going for just a hysterectomy or an exploratory operation and have come round to discover everything has 'been taken away'. Doctors' ignorance and arrogance has been a factor. In 1996 a doctor was struck off by the General Medical Council (GMC) after he removed a perfectly normal ovary at the Luton and Dunstable Hospital, even though the patient had insisted it should not be touched. Apparently, the doctor was told in the theatre that his patient was 'about 50' and he joked, 'She won't be needing these then, will she?' She was in fact 42.

In the early part of 2000, Caroline Richmond, a medical journalist from Battersea in south London, described feeling mutilated after she discovered her womb and ovaries had been removed during what she had believed to be an exploration into the cause of a prolonged period of heavy bleeding that had lasted for ten years. Her consultant, Mr Ian Fergusson, was found to have acted in good faith because, during the operation in 1992, he was concerned about a lump which he thought may have been malignant. The GMC committee reported that he had been medically justified in his actions, but he was criticised because 'the process of counselling the patient and obtaining her consent left a lot to be desired'.

Mrs Wendy Savage, the obstetrician and gynaecologist who came to prominence over her radical support of women's right to have their wishes taken into account over the way they give birth, appeared on Channel 4 news to discuss the Richmond case. She appeared to support the GMC's decision, pointing out that the incidents under review had taken place a long time ago and that, as a result of a number of questionable cases, consent forms are now required to take much more detailed account of a patient's wishes before surgery. She was, though, obviously outraged at the prophylactic removal of a woman's ovaries, without her permission having been expressly given.

'Imagine', she said, 'the outcry if a man had gone into hospital to have his gall bladder removed and the surgeon thought it would be a good idea, to prevent any future risk of testicular cancer, to cut off his balls.' Quite. So it is worth, unlike Sandy Chalmers, making sure you do ask lots of questions, informing yourself properly about what's intended if you have to have surgery and filling out the consent form with great care. Above all, make sure the surgeon who is to carry out the operation talks to you. Most conscientious ones do; but don't be fobbed off with some tired junior who won't finally be responsible for wielding the scalpel!

Some women don't have their menopause until they are in their late fifties, or, in some very rare cases, until 60. Excess body fat can delay menopause as oestrogen is produced in fatty tissues of the body, but this is not necessarily a good thing. An overabundance of circulating oestrogen is thought to increase the risk of some cancers – it's believed, for example, to be a factor in some breast and uterine cancers. Also, women who have diabetes may experience a later-than-average menopause, again because of higher levels of oestrogen. It's recommended that, if you are still menstruating in your late fifties, you should have a precautionary check-up with your GP.

Regardless of when it happens, there are profound changes to the body's chemistry during menopause which are measurable. (Scientific bit here!) The normal menstrual cycle, as we all know, results in a regular pattern of bleeding each month. One or other of the two ovaries releases an egg that travels down the Fallopian tube to the uterus. Before the egg is released, the lining of the womb, or endometrium, thickens ready to receive the egg, should it be fertilised by a sperm, and to nourish the embryonic pregnancy. If there is no conception the egg doesn't implant itself, the hormones that would support it diminish, the lining of the womb breaks down and is shed, and the whole process begins again.

It's the body's endocrine or glandular system that regulates the release of eggs, thousands of which are already present in the newborn baby girl, and the preparation of the womb lining. The system is controlled overall by the hypothalamus in the brain which can be disrupted by stress or drastic changes in body weight. This is why anorexia nervosa can cause periods to stop.

When the hypothalamus is in tip-top condition, it releases hormone messengers into the bloodstream regularly. These, in turn, stimulate the nearby pituitary gland to release its own hormone messengers, collectively known as gonadotrophins. GnRH is the gonadotrophin-releasing hormone and the two gonadotrophins are the follicle-stimulating hormone (FSH) and the luteinising hormone (LH).

The function of FSH is to stimulate the more mature egg follicles in the ovaries to produce another hormone, oestradiol, a form of oestrogen which in turn thickens the lining of the womb. When the oestradiol level reaches a peak it tells the hypothalamus to release more GnRH, which results in LH being secreted from the pituitary to the bloodstream. The LH acts on the most mature ovarian follicle, which bursts, releases the enclosed egg and completes the ovulation process.

The ruptured follicle that is left behind is known as the corpeus luteum. This produces oestradiol and the progesterone which helps to prepare the lining of the womb for the fertilised egg. If there is no pregnancy the hormone levels fall, the corpus luteum collapses, the lining breaks down and all of us who didn't want to be pregnant anyway breathe a sigh of relief as the period begins. Oestrogen levels fall, the pituitary gland cottons on, sends out another lot of FSH and the whole cycle begins again.

At the onset of the menopause there is a gradual reduction in the number of egg follicles in the ovaries. At birth, it's believed there are as many as 450,000 follicles in the ovaries. If ovulation begins on average at 12, at puberty, and ceases at around 52, at the menopause, only 500 ripened eggs have been released. During each menstrual cycle a number of follicles ripen at the same time, but only one releases an egg. The remainder become redundant. Others are thought to disappear gradually over the years, but there is still a dramatic loss of follicles (which can reach as few as 1000) once a woman reaches her forties. The reason for this remains a medical mystery.

As the supply of eggs in the ovaries dwindles, the eggs that remain become less responsive to the hormones which are secreted for their stimulation. Oestrogen levels fall, the pituitary gland recognises what's happening and each month frantically increases its production of FSH in an attempt to kick-start the reproductive system as normal.

As things progress and other symptoms such as flushes and sweats begin, blood levels of FSH rise significantly. As oestrogen levels fall because the egg follicles are not responding to FSH to produce it, LH rises to a level three to five times its normal premenstrual level. Blood tests for the increased presence of FSH is therefore useful in establishing whether a woman is peri-menopausal or not, usually when there are other symptoms present. (Bear in mind, though, that in the early part of the perimenopause, FSH levels can fluctuate, so having only one blood test may be misleading.) This hormonal tango explains why periods might become longer in duration, shorter, heavier or lighter or go into the stop-start mode so many of the women I've spoken to have described. As we've already seen, in some women – around 10 per cent – their periods will stop quickly and suddenly, while for others the inconvenience of an erratic cycle can go on for several years.

Although mature ovaries no longer ovulate, they do not cease to function entirely. The central region is actively engaged in producing the hormones testosterone and androstenedione which convert into oestrone, the form of oestrogen which remains circulating in the blood after the menopause. Testosterone, by the way, generally thought of as a male hormone, is an important influence on women's sexual arousal. Its production does not rise during the menopause, but it can become more dominant than in the past because levels of other hormones are falling. This could account for Melba Wilson's earlier description of her new-found, post-menopausal, humdinging multiple orgasms!

The down side of an increased dominance in testosterone levels can be the development of what are generally thought to be male characteristics. Around the menopause and after, some women notice an increased growth of facial hair and a deepening of the voice. For me, the former is one little hair on the right side of the chin – easily dealt with, using tweezers. Any more than that and I'll be off like a shot to the beauty parlour for epilation, where the hair is removed from the root with an electrical charge and shouldn't return. The deeper voice in my case is a professional bonus!

More supplies of oestrogen come from the adrenal glands and by processes in fat cells and from other extra-glandular sources. So, as the ovaries shut down, the body readjusts – substituting other oestrogen sources – although not in the same quantities as were produced during the normal menstrual cycle. In the first year after menopause the average drop in oestrogen level is 80 per cent.

It is estimated that 75 per cent to 80 per cent of women passing through menopause will experience one or more of the symptoms we've discussed, but only 10 per cent to 35 per cent say they were affected strongly enough to seek help and there is no consensus about how the severity of symptoms is affected by genetics, upbringing, culture, lifestyle or diet. Low menopausal distress has been associated with women who have never been married, never had children or had children late in life, and with higher levels of income and education. Ruth Lee, policy director at the Institute of Directors would suggest that none of these factors necessarily applies. She has never married, has no children, is highly educated and well paid, but at the age of 42 and working fiendishly long hours in a high-powered job as an economist in the City with a Japanese bank, she began to experience debilitating and embarrassing hot flushes – bad enough to send her to her doctor.

The highest levels of distress are said to be experienced by married women and mothers. It's not difficult to deduce that these circumstances may contribute to the symptoms, as worries about teenagers and juggling a relationship which may have hit the buffers of the 20-odd-year itch can't be underestimated, although the fitness instructor Penny Heeley bucks this trend, sailing through with barely a symptom, a husband and a son. There seem to be few hard-and-fast guidelines, although women who have suffered painful periods and severe premenstrual syndrome in the past and those who have undergone premature menopause, either natural or surgical, are said to report a particularly bad time. This, too, on the basis of my conversations with women who do not fit these profiles, but had horrendous symptoms, may be too much of a generalisation to give any help to you if you're not menopausal yet and looking for predictions. Wait and see is, I think, the best policy.

The great debate is, of course, the degree to which menopausal symptoms can be linked to falling oestrogen levels. Proponents of hormone replacement therapy (HRT) will often argue that the link is undisputed. Oestrogen does, indeed, have a huge effect on female physical health. Apart from its direct action on the uterus as part of the reproductive system, it is said to influence other organs and tissues such as the vagina (as we've already discussed), vulva, breasts, heart, hair, skin, central nervous system and bones. The most commonly feared result of menopause is osteoporosis – a reduction in bone density which can cause frequent breaks, stooping and lameness.

Jo Wagerman – at 67 the first woman to be elected chairman of the British Board of Jewish Deputies – feared menopause because both her mother and grandmother had developed a dowager's hump by the time they were 50 and, by 60, walked stiffly with a stick – both direct results of osteoporosis. Jo was terrified that she, too, would end up in the same position, bowed and frequently in plaster after breaking her limbs. She was a teacher before retirement and all she wanted, she says, was to be able to continue standing up straight. She is convinced of a direct correlation between oestrogen deficiency and the bone disease.

Much medical literature focuses on the effect oestrogen plays in every organ of the body and the changes said to be inevitable as it falls. Robert Wilson, an American gynaecologist and author, published *Feminine Forever* in 1966, and is often quoted by those who see the menopause and life after as a deficient state. He described the menopause as 'living decay, a destruction of personality and an aberration'. The menopause in his view is a serious, painful and often crippling disease, leading in its worst manifestation to suicide. Commentators who followed him, such as Dr David Reuben, author of *Everything You Wanted to Know About Sex*, Wendy Cooper, the journalist who wrote *No Change* and, most recently, Dr Miriam Stoppard, in her book *Menopause*, shared Wilson's enthusiasm for hormone replacement to 'cure this deficiency disease'. (There'll be more details about attitudes to treatments over the years in Chapter 2).

So from the medical evidence we have to hand, how much can really be put down to oestrogen deficiency? It is widely believed that oestrogen plays a part in the development, post-menopausally, of osteoporosis. Women are more likely than men to be prone to low bone density and this decreases measurably after the menopause. (We'll talk about the arguments for and against bone density tests in Chapter 3.) A third of all adult women will suffer at least one osteoporotic fracture in their lifetime. As people grow older, the process of bone renewal slows down through natural ageing and various factors, such as nutrition, exercise and genetics, can affect the risk of future fractures, but oestrogen is generally accepted to be responsible for maintaining bone mass and helping with the constant process of bone renewal. When levels of the hormone fall, less calcium is directed at and absorbed into the bones.

Hot flushes, night sweats and palpitations are linked to the endocrine system. It is thought that the hypothalamus in the brain, which, as we've seen, orchestrates many of our hormonal functions, also influences the body's temperature control and circulation of the blood. Blood vessels dilate, increasing flow to the skin and raising its temperature. That's when we get the sudden sensation of overwhelming heat. Then we sweat, which leads to a rapid cooling. As the temperature increases so sometimes does the pulse, hence the occasional sensation of palpitations which can accompany hot flushes and night sweats. This is the 'Yes it's me, it isn't hot in here' syndrome!

Falling progesterone levels – caused because the changing reproductive system no longer needs this particular hormone to prepare the uterus for pregnancy – has only recently been recognised as a potentially crucial factor. Decreasing levels of progesterone before and during menopause may exacerbate symptoms of oestrogen excess such as heavy and erratic periods. (More details on this in Chapters 4, 5 and 6.)

In those women who do report vaginal dryness there may be a hormonal link. Oestrogen deficiency is said to cause the vagina to become shorter and less elastic, although another common cause is post-hysterectomy, where some of the mucus-secreting glands may have been destroyed. Most of us, however, can fix this problem if we have it. I've already mentioned the benefits of a rich fantasy life, imaginative, thoughtful and informed lovers, pelvic floor exercises and the fact that putting the vagina to its intended use from time to time will help to keep it lubricated as well. Other tips include avoiding irritating soaps, scented oils and bubble baths. You should wear cotton knickers to help to prevent itching and infection. In Chapter 5 we'll examine claims for the efficacy of oestrogen cream applied directly to the area.

Urinary incontinence is something lots of us have suffered – and there's nothing more embarrassing than trying to conceal a wet patch on your leotard during an aerobics class. For most of us it's the result of childbirth and a cavalier attitude, post-natally, to the pelvic floor. The good news is it ain't too late to start doing exercises now (details later). There is evidence of a connection between loss of oestrogen and some sagging in the structures which support the bladder. Again, exercise is useful. Nicotine, caffeine and diet pills are thought to make incontinence worse, as is the pressure on the lower regions caused by being excessively overweight. If the problem is really ruining your life there is, as a last resort, corrective surgery that can help. I've found that going to the loo when I first feel the urge is the best policy. It's not necessarily more frequent than in the past, unless I've consumed more than a sensible dose of coffee. We've all been used, since we were little girls, to putting it off, primarily because of the dearth of toilets when we're out and about. Assuming you can hold it in becomes a more risky business with age. Golden rule: if there's a loo available, use it, whether you think you want to or not – you'll find you do when you get there.

Where dry or itchy skin, thinning hair or pins and needles are reported the precise cause is not known. Skin becomes thinner as it loses collagen, its main support structure, and becomes less elastic. The loss of collagen is more rapid in the first few years after the menopause and 30 per cent of skin collagen is lost within the first five years. The rate of decrease is approximately 2 per cent per year for the first ten years. This is thought to be caused by a combination of natural ageing, environmental and hormonal factors. Some women have hair loss; others, as mentioned earlier, find their hair is more abundant, and this is most likely to be influenced by changing levels of oestrogen and testosterone. A feeling called 'formication', which derives from the Latin word for ant, is sometimes complained of and described as 'ants crawling over the skin'. No one can pin down a reason for this.

Most of us also notice some joint and muscle pains and a bit of a sag around the chin line. The breasts, as the comedian Joan Rivers put it, rush to meet the ground, and the waistline and pelvic floor begin to lose their tone. Exercise and a sense of humour are probably the most useful tools in combating these developments. Muscles are affected by testosterone and, although it may become more dominant relative to oestrogen, falling levels may be a factor. In his book, *A Change for the Better*, Dr Hilary Jones quotes studies where HRT in post-menopausal women has shown a significant increase in muscle tone and some of the HRT devotees I've spoken to report improvements in their skin once they start taking the tablets (more details in Chapter 5).

Painful and lumpy breasts are a common complaint during menopause – I'll tell you later, in Chapter 3 (p. 75), about the ghastly scare I had after a dodgy mammogram and eventually found what turned out to be nothing more serious than totally benign cysts. Fibrocystic disease affects a large percentage of women and can be very scary. Any lump we always assume to be cancer, although frequently it's not. Although some doctors believe there may be a link between breast cysts and oestrogen, a US research study suggests no connection and shows that they can be eliminated in 80 per cent of cases by a change in lifestyle. Giving up smoking, caffeine and chocolate and taking a supplement of vitamin E each day are the recommended strategies.

Weight gain and the redistribution of body fat is something most of us – unless we are the kind of fit Penny Heeley can boast – will experience. Extra fatty tissue tends to settle in the abdominal area and we will all become more apple- and less pear-shaped. This may be connected with falling oestrogen, although some women report dramatic weight gain as a result of HRT (see Chapter 5). More likely is a fall in metabolic rate which is common to both men and women in mid-life and too much time spent sitting on the sofa watching TV and eating chocolate!

The journalist and broadcaster Joan Bakewell says she often sees her weight creeping up half a stone and when she starts to feel uncomfortable she eats less as it's the only way to keep herself at a healthy weight as she's got older.

Headaches and migraines may be hormonal or not. Headaches may become more common because of tension, stress and worry. Teenage children, needy adult relatives, the pressures of keeping on top of a job, worries about husbands or partners who may be roaming as a result of their own mid-life crisis, or concerns about poverty in middle age for women who are alone and may be short of pension funds, are all extremely stressful.

Constipation and irritable bowel syndrome are sometimes exacerbated at this time and there is some evidence to suggest that hormones may play a part in intestinal movement. Reduced physical activity and normal changes to the pelvic organs caused by the ageing process also have an effect.

Psychological problems are, as we've seen, experienced by a significant number of women, regardless of their age at menopause, but there is passionate disagreement about whether they can be put down to hormonal changes or not. We may wrongly attribute them to the menopause, as may doctors, many of whom are now in the habit of seeing menopause as a medical disaster area. Dr Miriam Stoppard says that the centres of the brain that control a sense of well-being, a positive state of mind and a feeling of control and tranquillity are affected by the absence of oestrogen, as are memory, conceptual thinking and perception. 'Some of the effects of oestrogen are as therapeutic as those of tranquillisers and, in a way, menopausal women are suffering from "natural tranquilliser withdrawal".'

The most recent research from the United States would seem to back up this theory. Studies are said to show that oestrogen receptors are abundant in the brain and that oestrogen has a role in many brain processes such as cerebral blood flow, glucose administration, synaptic activity and neuronal growth, as well as complex functions such as cognition. In general, then, it is said that oestrogen has a positive effect on mood and contributes to a sense of well-being, although the role of oestrogen deficiency in serious post-menopausal depression, declining cognitive function, dementia and Alzheimer's disease is not clear and is still an area of intensive debate and research (see Chapter 5).

For example, one study which found a positive correlation between perimenopause and depressive symptoms acknowledged that a prior history of depression may have been a factor. Another found hardly any difference between men and women in the clarity of their thought processes as they aged although full Alzheimer's is more common in women by a ratio of 3:1. The most recent study, published in August 2000, claimed that women were marginally less able to carry out complex tasks than men of the same middle age. Researchers pointed to the fact that the women appeared capable of concentrating on only one job at a time. This, in my experience, is what men have always found – but at least when we were younger we were used to juggling a million balls in the air. If there is any truth in this recent research, it could be seen as a useful function of the menopause, allowing us finally to be as single-minded as men are able to be, and letting us off the hook of having to worry about the dinner, the dog, the dusting and the demanding job.

This was not, of course, the spin put on the research by British newspapers which reported it. They were universally negative in their analysis of its meaning. There have been numerous occasions where the press have leaped on the findings of such research, too many times to be dismissed as insignificant. The American journalist Susan Faludi analysed newspaper coverage in the 1990s and found a concerted campaign to keep women in their place, for which she coined the title, 'the Backlash'. So we should be extremely wary of research which is carried out over a short period of time, using a small sample (in this case only 60) of women which suggests that women are less capable than men and is given extensive newpaper coverage.

In her book *No Change* Wendy Cooper pointed to studies with

WHAT IS THE MENOPAUSE?   37

depression being linked to lack of oestrogen and quotes a British doctor, John Studd, who told her he has been using oestrogen implants for years to treat various forms of female depression, including that linked to the menopause. Others disagree, saying depression or 'feeling a bit down' can have other physical or social causes (and we all know men who go a bit peculiar at this age, don't we?) What is important to be aware of is that, whether or not you choose to treat the feelings of misery when they are at their most acute, it is very unusual for these miseries to last. Women past the age of the menopause have no more depression than men of the same age.

The official view of the North American Menopause Society is as follows:

Among the many myths associated with menopause is that mental health problems such as depression and anxiety are inevitable as hormone production decreases. In reality, there are no scientific studies to support the belief that natural menopause is responsible for true clinical depression, anxiety, severe memory lapses or erratic behaviour. However, many mid-life women do suffer from feeling blue, discouraged, irritable and tired. Women deserve answers to get them through difficult times so they can thrive during what can be the best years of their lives. Most women become accustomed to their own hormonal rhythm during their reproductive years. During the perimenopause, the rhythm changes. The hormone fluctuations, though normal, can still be stress-provoking. Many women find the unexpected timing and extent of these changes create upset and a sense of loss of control. For some women, the hormone-related changes coincide with other stressors and losses.

Eyesight diminishes in both men and women at around the age of 45. My optician tells me this is because of drying in the lens, which can no longer expand and contract in response to light sources as it has in the past. Thus, reading and close work become more difficult, whereas distance vision takes longer to be affected. It is, she says, because the eye is the only organ in the body which has failed to evolve to accommodate greater life expectancy. There is some new evidence to show a possible link between falling oestrogen levels and some vision-threatening conditions in post-menopausal women which predominantly affect us over the age of 60. It is always advisable to have your eyes checked regularly for diseases such as glaucoma, which, with early detection, can be successfully treated. Otherwise you just have to learn to live with specs. I've managed to adopt mine as part of my character. When I peer over them at interviewees who fail fully to answer my questions, strong politicians are said to tremble with fright!

Coronary heart disease (CHD) is the biggest single killer of post-menopausal women. Proponents of HRT believe that oestrogen protects women from heart disease by reducing the bad cholesterol (LDL) and increasing good cholesterol (HDL). Oestrogen is also believed to increase the production of a substance which relaxes the walls of the blood vessels and helps to keep coronary arteries wide open. It is also said to inhibit another substance that is associated with hardening of the arteries and heart attacks. This contention is hotly debated. Several researchers have said that there has been selection bias in the studies which have been carried out so far and that women in the trials may already have been healthier than the average. Those in favour say the results are impressive, even taking into account this question mark over the efficacy of the trials. There are also questions to be considered about the effect of progestogens on CHD, which may counter any beneficial effects of oestrogen. (There'll be more about this in Chapter 5.)

Menopause itself has not been directly associated with any increased risk of cancer, but cancer rates do typically increase with age, so women in midlife and beyond need to be aware of cancer of the lung (especially if they smoke), breast, uterus, ovary, colon, rectum and skin – the most common cancers affecting women. Approximately 80 per cent of breast cancers appear in women who are post-menopausal, although the jury is still out on the influence of oestrogen in all cancers of the breast and reproductive organs and it should be remembered that middle-aged women who do suffer from breast cancer tend to have the slower growing type of tumour for which treatments are now very effective.

It's becoming apparent that there may well be other biological processes going on in the body, in addition to hormonal changes, which may produce some of the common symptoms we've talked about and that there are health issues to which we should pay attention as we get older which have absolutely nothing to do with the menopause. Aches and pains could indeed be rheumatism or arthritis. Fatigue might be a post-viral syndrome or a thyroid disorder. Depression, anxiety and insomnia may well be due to other factors – worrying about children leaving the nest, how to hang on to a job or a partner, whether the pension will be enough to keep us in our old age or, as Linda Taylor, the 50-year-old post-menopausal member of the girl band Six Chicks, puts it, 'Whether I'll be a woman any more or whether I'll turn out like a dried-up crisp. Will I ever work in this business again?' All these things need to be thought about and discussed, rather than making the assumption that it's 'bound to be yer 'ormones, dear!' (see Chapter 3).

In *The Change*, Germaine Greer challenges the assumption that oestrogen deficiency causes climacteric symptoms:

It has never been substantiated by empirical proof, despite the best efforts of an army of clinicians and biochemists supported by the vast resources of pharmaceutical multinationals. The usual account makes it seem only ovulation and menstruation can keep women feeling well. This is not what a young woman herself

*perceived when, after 14 years or so of feeling as well as can be,
menstruation suddenly made her feel sick . . . the obstacle to
understanding here is the defect that disfigures all gynaecological
investigation; we do not know enough about the well woman to
understand what has gone wrong with the sick one.*

As I have discovered in some of my interviews, notably with
Glenda Jackson and Penny Heeley, some women go through the
menopause with no symptoms at all or a minimum of inconvenience and we have not yet identified the mechanism which
makes these women different from the majority who do seem to
suffer. But even though they seem to be in a lucky minority, their
very existence would suggest that menopause could be viewed as a
natural process and not a signal of disease which necessarily
requires medical treatment.

In another e-mail, my friend Griselda summed up what I hope
this chapter has uncovered and what this whole book is about. A
search for a better understanding of what is happening to us
physically, what we can do about it and how we can learn to make
informed decisions about the best way to act as regards the medical
profession, friends, children and partners. Primarily, though, I
hope that through sharing our experiences of what we suffer or not,
as the case may be, we find some comfort in the fact that we are not
alone, that there are various strategies for making ourselves feel
better and that these feelings will not go on for ever. Here's what
she wrote.

*In an analytical frame of mind, one impression is that symptoms
are bearable on the way 'up' to the menopause itself (has it
happened yet? I don't know, do I?). But things go seriously and
dreadfully wrong and much, much worse on the way down.
(Perhaps one should think of it as a valley to cross rather than a hill
to climb.) The mental impairment, the doubt, the loss of*

understanding of stuff – that's what's so frightening. 'Hot flushes' comes nowhere near describing what it feels like. My mother is dead, and so is her sister Flora, who might have told me something about how women in our family deal with this. All I can do is talk out loud about what I think has been completely taboo in public. I tell the gobsmacked men and women that I am menopausal. I say I'm hot, I don't understand, I'm tired. I explain it is a special spiritual rite of passage, a beginning of a world of understanding they know nothing of. I am even more difficult, exasperating and unreliable than usual and that's because I am becoming MORE IMPORTANT. Sometimes I believe it, too. Mostly it's hard graft.

CHAPTER 2

HOW THE MENOPAUSE
BECAME A BATTLEGROUND

In a frequent exchange of e-mails on the subject of our own woes, unanswered questions, doubts and irritations at the failure of the wider world to begin to sympathise with or comprehend the reality of our experiences at the time of the menopause and after, another old pal of mine expressed her fury with a doctor.

> Yesterday I finally went to a doc to ask for HRT. I asked him, 'What is the purpose of the climacteric?' and he thought for a while and said, 'Women were not designed to live this long.' (I felt incandescent with rage at this, and simultaneously wanted to die.) I said, 'What about grandmothers, tribal memory, respect for elders, etc?' He said, speculatively, 'No other primates have a menopause, so humans shouldn't.' I said, 'Gimme the patch, doc.' But there still remains the question. What is the purpose of the climacteric? I can only think of babies' teething pain as an equivalent: something to signal to the wider group that an important change is taking place.

She is not alone in her irritation at the frequently dismissive and thoughtless attitudes of the medical profession and the lack of seriousness with which such an important time in a woman's life is generally treated. Lesley Hilton, a freelance journalist who specialises in medicine, health and social affairs, says that what gets her down is this idea of a lack of purpose in suffering all these symptoms. She's 48 and in the throes of her worst symptoms as I write. She's acutely aware of the problems hot flushes, feeling generally lethargic and fed-up and like a 'cantankerous old bag' are causing her. She recalls that when she was a teenager she felt bizarre, as she did when she was pregnant, but in both cases there seemed to be a positive outcome on the horizon. Menopause seems to have no real point, apart from making her wonder what she will be like as she ages – and the prospect, to her at least, appears not very hopeful.

She feels this is because we have none of the support systems for menopause that we had at earlier times in our lives. There are easily accessible antenatal groups, self-help for those with multiple births, miscarriage or neo-natal death, but menopause is still either swept under the carpet, dismissed as bordering on lunacy and consequently shameful, or seen only as a medical problem to be quickly fixed with pharmaceuticals.

She cites the scene of two pregnant women standing at the check-out in a supermarket. It's inconceivable that they would not comment to each other on their state of health or comfort, but she has never, she says, had a hot flush in the shops and found other women of the same age doing anything other than looking away in embarrassment. I have to say, I think this is changing, but slowly. (Just say 'Is it it me or is it hot in here?' – and see what response you get!)

Lesley was encouraged when she went to see her GP about another matter and saw an advertisement for a Menopause Group. She went along, hoping for conversation and shared experiences, and found there was no time for chatter or discussion of options. They were simply shown a video that had been prepared by a drug company, extolling the virtues of HRT. She thought it was a wholly inadequate response.

It is surprising that the women's movement has concerned itself with every other aspect of women's lives, but has failed to demand or establish informed networks for women in mid life. (See Useful Addresses for information on the newly formed Pennell Initiative for Women's Health and other contacts.) Perhaps it is understandable, as mine is the first generation to have come through the women's movement in the wake of its early pioneers and to benefit from their questions about the assumptions of the past. Women like Germaine Greer and Gloria Steinem, the second-wave feminists, are only now in their sixties, so it's perhaps not so astonishing that it's the third wave of third agers who are in a position to assess what ageing really means for us, what choices we have and what kind of demands we can make, in the light of the experiences we've watched them go through.

It is, of course, nonsense for a doctor to suggest that women were not designed to live this long. Lindsay Allison Jones, an expert on the Ancient Romans, says that the oldest recorded Roman female living in Britain was 90. It's obvious that more of us live to older ages now than in the past – childbirth is less hazardous, child mortality has fallen, medicine has made advances and even the working classes can expect to work, rest and play. But even in the mid 1680s, when the average life expectancy was 32, the middle and upper classes could expect to live much longer, as their diet and home life was better and they were not forced to work relentlessly from dawn till dusk in dangerous, unhealthy conditions. The historian Michael Anderson has calculated that of those born in Britain in 1681, 18 per cent of men and 21 per cent of women were still alive at 53. In English villages, 10 per cent of the inhabitants were 60 or more.

Among the wealthy, those who survived until they came of age, at 21, could expect, on average, to live well into their sixties –

indeed, most European countries considered men fit for military
service until they were 60. Women could expect even longer lives
in the upper classes. Since official registration began, it has been
obvious that women, as long as they survived childbirth, have
traditionally lived longer than men. In her book *The Weaker
Vessel*, Antonia Fraser gives lots of examples of 17th-century
Englishwomen who lived into their nineties and beyond. There
have always been plenty of older women around, it's just that we
haven't heard about them.

There are a number of notable historical references in the
medical text books. In Ancient Egyptian papyruses post-menopausal women are indicated as white, in contrast with the younger,
fertile females who are shown as red. Aristotle observed that
women were unable to bear children after the age of 50, while a
sixth-century Byzantine doctor, Aecio de Amida, noted that
menstrual blood stopped at around the age of 50. The ancient
commentators influenced the medieval. In the 13th century,
Albertus Magnus followed Aristotle's observation that women
lived longer than men. He put it down to the fact that
menstruation purified women of harmful humours, that sexual
intercourse took away fewer of their bodily fluids, and that they
suffered less from the hazards of work (that to include war, no
doubt).

A new age in geriatric medicine began in the 15th century with
Paracelsus, who experimented with drugs derived from herbs,
minerals and other substances. Anatomy was studied by Vesalius
and Benevieni and Leonardo da Vinci carried out dissections on
elderly bodies and made observations. It was primarily men who
were studied, as women were rarely in a position to consult a
doctor, who would inevitably be a man, and the poor, whether
male or female, couldn't afford it, but at least some research was
done.

In 16th-century Europe the physicians who followed Galen

believed that women became more like men as they passed the menopause, becoming leaner, drier, and warmer than in earlier life and thus more likely to outlive their menfolk. Post-menopausal women were perceived as fitter, healthier and less threatening than younger women. Some, however, saw the end of menstruation – thought to be a purifier of the body – as a poisoning of women's bodies, leading to fornication and crime. It's interesting that the sexually voracious older woman, free from the risk of becoming pregnant, is still a 20th-century fear. Vera Ivers, chair of the Older Woman's Network, remembers her first husband – the one who was around when she had her hysterectomy in her late thirties – expressing the opinion that it would make her a loose woman. Even her mother asked her, when it became obvious her marriage was breaking down, 'You're not like *that* are you?'

In the 18th century, Titius published a thesis at the University of Magdeburg called *Cessation Menstruorum*. Thirty years later, the English doctor, Quincy, published a work in which he speaks for the first time of 'climax' in the sense of 'crisis' in the life of women. The term 'menopause' was only used a century later in 1816, when a French doctor, A. L. Gardanne, wrote of 'la menopausie' in *Avis aux femmes qui entrent dans l'âge critique*. It first appeared in this country under the heading 'Climacteric Insanity' in 1899 in an article on 'Epochal Insanities' contributed by a Dr Coulston to *A System of Medicine* by Many Writers.

It's only in our own time that large numbers of female historians and scholars have been in a position to show an interest in their own kind and to research and publish their findings. Pat Thane, the author of *Old Age in English History*, points to Euripides' representation of an older woman in Alcemene, the wife of Iolaus.

Compared with other characters, including Iolaus himself, she is defined by her strength and wrath, in contrast to the deference of the younger women. She is active, wielding power and authority in

contrast to her husband's weak dependence. Equally assertive older
women appear elsewhere in Greek literature: for example Hecuba
towards the end of the Iliad.

In *The Change*, Germaine Greer, searches for references to menopause in literature and, whilst she comes up with a number of older
female characters, such as sad, poor Miss Bates in Jane Austen's
Emma or silly Mrs Bennett in *Pride and Prejudice*, they are generally
made fun of. Elizabeth Gaskell wrote *Cranford* when she had just
turned 40 herself; nevertheless it's dottiness that is the prime
characteristic of Miss Matty, who, in a rare literary moment,
admits her age is 52. She is already dithery and forgetful, and
sometimes wears one cap on top of another. Greer writes:

> *A hundred pages later Miss Matty cannot walk very fast; she has*
> *a touch of rheumatism and her eyes are failing. In case we should*
> *console ourselves with the thought that old people get younger with*
> *every generation that passes and 50 year olds are younger and*
> *spryer now than they were then, we are brought up short by Miss*
> *Matty saying, 'We are principally ladies now I know, but we are*
> *not so old as ladies used to be when I was a girl.'*

Greer also says that, since she became interested in women over
50, she has turned to biographies and memoirs, searching for the
moment of change, but she has found very little. This is partly
because women who may have been in a position to record their
experience, such as Mary Wollstonecraft or Charlotte Brontë, died
in childbirth or as a consequence of miscarriage, infectious disease
or epidemic. Greer believes that the ones who did survive into
menopause and beyond chose not to discuss it, even in an encoded
fashion, because to appear in print was to expose oneself in mixed
company and the menopause was no more likely to be mentioned
than any other female bodily function.

Even the 18th-century novelist and playwright, Fanny Burney, makes no mention of her menopause in her extensive diaries, although she does give a most detailed and horrific description of the mastectomy she underwent in France after she was diagnosed with breast cancer. She lived for another 20 fruitful years after the radical surgery, into her eighties. Greer is convinced that this lack of shared experience – a silence, even on the part of the most articulate and noisy women of the past – contributes greatly to our fear and anxiety of the menopause and its aftermath.

Greer does mention one woman whose menopause she managed to detect through learning to interpret what few signs there are. In 1818 one Maria Edgeworth is said to have been severely depressed and suffered 'alarming weakness of her eyes'. Both, says Greer, are usually explained as a result of family troubles and the worry that she might contract serious illness in her dealings with the Irish peasantry, but take on a more meaningful significance when we discover that, in that year, Maria turned 51. Her doctor is said to have been most alarmed and prescribed a period of enforced inactivity. Maria gave up reading, writing and needlework for two years and then recovered.

Sixteen years later she was well enough to tour Connemara and began to learn Spanish at the age of 70. Jane Austen sent her a copy of *Emma*; she received 150 barrels of flour from Boston for her relief work during the Irish famine and was said to be extremely lively until she was 82, when she died peacefully in the arms of her close friend and her father's fourth wife, Frances Beaufort.

The idea that menopause equals lunacy, danger or sheer nastiness goes back a long way. In medieval times, as we've seen, it was a commonly held belief that menopausal disturbances happened because menstruation no longer discharged bad humours from the womb. There was grave concern that the end of menstrual flow led to the development of dangerous symptoms. It was never considered to signify a natural process, freeing women from their fertility, and this thinking persisted into the 19th century. If we think we've got it tough, we don't know we're born compared with women who sought medical treatment in those days.

Bloodletting was frequently prescribed to purge and cleanse the body of excess and impure blood. Practices included deliberately opening wounds or veins and administering leeches – sometimes (and you didn't really want to know this!) to the cervix – ouch! Other treatments included the prescription of herbal remedies – Agnus Castus is still in use for menstrual imbalances – purgatives, and taking the waters in spa towns and cities such as Buxton or Bath. Occasionally doctors would even recommend the ingestion of toxic metals, including lead, which can't have done anyone any good.

Medical literature of the late 18th century refers to the menopause as a catastrophic attack and tragedy, with post-menopausal women being described as dull and unattractive. During the early part of the 19th century, doctors believed that normal menstrual blood was being disposed of by haemorrhages or hot flushes and after the menopause the blood that was no longer expelled turned to fat. (I have a curious attraction to this particular theory – it can't just be greed and a sedentary lifestyle that's led to this spreading of the waistline, can it?!)

A more systematic interest in the menopause by medical professionals began in the mid-19th century. At that time, the medical profession was all male. Elizabeth Garret Anderson was the first qualified woman to practise in the UK, having gained her medical degree abroad in 1865. Before her, the only woman to have worked as a doctor in Britain was James Miranda Barry, who studied at Edinburgh and was appointed an army surgeon in 1813. She spent her entire career, both as a student and as a professional, disguised as a man, so she can't have been much help in furthering enlightenment about the menopause, although she lived to be 70 and presumably had one. One wonders how she explained a hot flush to her colleagues in the mess. In her book *Menopause and Culture*, Gabriella Berger writes that:

> In Victorian England, medical advertisements and writings reveal an obsession of the medical profession with female secretions, particularly those of menstruation. The perception that the menopause causes disease was quite prominent at that time and opened the door to medical intervention.
>
> Menopause was seen as a sensitive physiological turning point in a woman's life, a developmental crisis. A painful or depressed puberty was held to be responsible for a traumatic menopause and both milestones were described by an eminent 19th-century physician as 'the two termini of a woman's sexual activity'. It was thought a woman's life was dictated by her ovaries. Doctors also contended that the female body contained a limited amount of energy, all of which was needed for the development of the uterus and the ovaries. Menopausal women were said to struggle to overcome this partial death, this biological withering and their decreased sexual desire.

During this time, menopause was also linked with psychological problems: anxiety, sleeplessness and hot flushes were often treated as hysteria, that curiously female condition invented by Hippocrates who believed the womb (in Greek, *hustera*) had an energy all its own and a powerful hold over women. His misunderstanding, all those years ago, has a great deal to answer for.

For some medical practitioners, the menopause represented the death throes of the womb and even at the start of the 20th century was held responsible for all manner of ills, including tuberculosis, diabetes, depression and insanity. A woman who suffered menopausal symptoms was thought to have only herself to blame. As Dr Anne McGregor writes:

Support for the suffragette movement was cited as a cause for severe menopausal symptoms; indeed any woman who was too highly educated, indulged in an undue amount of sex or showed insufficient devotion to her husband and children was bound to suffer.

The recommended treatment followed similar misconceptions. Women were supposed to avoid any sexual excitement at the menopause, since it might attract blood to the brain. If menstrual blood did manage to enter the brain it would trigger mental symptoms, hot flushes and perspiration. Fortunately, the picture of the menopause was not always gloomy. Some doctors had a more enlightened approach; they saw menopause as 'the Indian summer of a woman's life' – a time of extra energy, optimism and beauty.

One of the more enlightened according to Germaine Greer was Edward John Tilt, a fashionable ladies' doctor who worked in London from 1850. He wrote a book called *The Change of Life in Health* in 1857 which he based – rarely for his time, as, indeed, today – on conversations with his female patients about their experience of the menopause. He accepted that the menopause was brought about by real, not imagined, physical changes in the body and described it as 'a beautiful series of critical movements – the object of which is to endow a woman with a greater degree of strength than she previously enjoyed'.

Tilt believed the processes of the menopause were as natural as the processes of adolescence and childbirth and saw his job as helping a woman through this difficult time with a minimum of suffering. At the conclusion of the menopause, he observed, mature women were less likely to contract infectious illnesses than younger women and had greater powers of endurance than those who were still going through menstruation, pregnancy and child-birth. He saw a role for older women as the guardians of young mothers and the arbiters of taste and good manners.

The first connection between symptoms and the cessation of ovarian function was made at the turn of the 19th and 20th centuries. The first recorded attempt to treat women with ovarian therapy was in Berlin in 1896, and the therapies prescribed were, naturally, unpleasant. The choices on offer were extract of placenta, the urine of pregnant women, fresh ovarian juice or extracts of ovaries (I can't find out how it was extracted and, frankly, it doesn't bear thinking about), or powdered ovaries, made up as a tablet to be taken orally or implanted.

In the 1920s the science of endocrinology began to take off. In 1923 and 1929, respectively, the hormones oestrogen and progesterone were identified, but still could not be used easily as treatments. When taken by mouth, natural human hormones are rendered inactive by digestive juices, so the only method of administration was by injection. Oestrogen from animal sources, which, it was thought, could be ingested, was first isolated from the urine of pregnant mares, as it still is today.

By the 1940s scientists had produced synthetic versions of natural hormones which could be taken orally and Premarin, one of the most widely used HRT pharmaceuticals, was developed from mares' urine. By 1945, full-page advertisements for it were appearing in the *American Journal of Obstetrics and Gynaecology*. It was used to a limited extent by consultants in the US and Britain in the 1940s and 1950s, although there was uncertainty about risks and benefits. In the 1940s the connection was made between osteoporosis and oestrogen deficiency and the demand for prescriptions increased significantly.

I have it from two separate, informed and reliable sources that the Queen Mum was one of the first to try HRT and the timing is right. She would have become menopausal in the late 1940s and she is said to have continued with it ever since. If it is true, and I have no reason to disbelieve my informants, she's a jolly good advert, walking down the steps and into her car unaided as she did during her hundredth birthday celebrations and with a skin quality that certainly belies her great age.

After the contraceptive pill was developed using synthetic hormones, it was made available in the US in 1960. Scare stories about the increased risk of thrombosis, heart disease and stroke as a result of taking the pill quickly began to circulate and again by association, the safety of HRT came under scrutiny. Research at the time suggested that the lower dose of natural oestrogens in HRT, far from adding to the risk, could in fact protect against heart disease.

It was Robert Wilson, a British-born gynaecologist working in New York, who can be credited with the beginnings of mass usage of HRT. In the 1950s and 1960s, he began to push the theory that replacing oestrogen could eliminate menopausal symptoms and he treated many thousands of women, administering the treatment first by injection and later orally. He also kept up a flow of medical papers and articles on the subject and set up the Wilson Foundation, dedicated to funding, partly through drug companies, and inspiring research and the dessemination of information about the benefits of HRT.

Robert Wilson published his book, *Feminine Forever*, in 1966, with the intention of popularising HRT (or ERT – estrogen replacement therapy, as it's known in the States), and sure enough, women hungry for information and comfort bought 100,000 copies in the first seven months after it first arrived in the bookshops. Respected women's magazines such as *Vogue* welcomed his analysis without criticism.

Wilson hailed oestrogen as the long sought elixir of life and called it 'the youth pill'. He advocated 'adequate oestrogen from puberty to grave' in order to eliminate the menopause. He described menopausal women as castrated by the menopause which was 'a serious, painful and often crippling disease'. Menopause, he opined, was an abnormal state of being and he listed up to 26 symptoms including absent-mindedness, irritability, depression and frigidity. He spoke of cases where 'the resulting physical and mental anguish was so unbearable that the patient committed suicide . . . no woman can be sure of escaping the horror of this living decay.' (No mention anywhere, you'll note, of balding, paunchy, creaking middle-aged men and their own 'living decay'! What a pity our reproductive lives have brought us so much more frequently into the clutches of the medics and exposed us to these calumnies. Men, who have to be dragged screaming to a doctor, generally preferring to moan at home, have escaped attention and remained free of these insults. So, hurray for those who're now beginning to identify a male menopause – now, perhaps, they'll know how it feels.)

Wilson went on to see 'desexed' women everywhere:

Once the veil is lifted it is remarkable how quickly the previously uninitiated can detect these unfortunate women. Our streets abound with them, walking stiffly in twos and threes, seeing little and observing less. It is not unusual to see an erect man of 75 striding along the golf course, but never a woman of this age **[Author's fury bursts through here! Tell this nonsense to Dame Alicia Markova – still the upright ballerina at 90, the Queen Mum, the choreographer Gillian Lynne still dancing in her seventies. I could go on and I shouldn't interrupt, but this guy makes me so mad! Still, it's important to know how we arrived at our current situation, so forgive me, but I'll allow him to go on.]** *Before this moderately advanced age is reached, the more intelligent woman instinctively knows that her loss of physical attractiveness is entire out of proportion. She sees the marked skin changes, the disfiguring fat deposits, the atrophy of her breasts and the beginning disappearance of her external genitals* **[Oh, yeah!!! Sorry! Interrupting again.]** *If married, an irritated or inadequate vagina* *may bring more unhappiness. All this has a profound effect on her psyche.*

I have seen untreated women who have shrivelled into caricatures of their former selves. Some had lost as much as six inches in height due to pathological bone changes caused by lack of oestrogen [**Author's note again – men lose height, too, due to the ageing process, so this is a bit of an exaggeration.**] *Others suffered sweeping metabolic disturbances that literally put them in mortal danger. Though the physical symptoms can be truly dreadful, what impresses me most tragically is the destruction of personality. Some women when they realise they are no longer women subside into a stupor of indifference. Even so they are relatively lucky. The most heart-breaking cases I feel are those sensitive women who witness their own decline with agonising self-awareness.*

And, guess what? He blames his mum for this bitter and poisonous view of the maturing woman. He says as a teenager he witnessed her going through the unmentionable 'change of life'.

I was appalled by the transformation of the vital wonderful woman who had been the dynamic focal point of our family into a pain-wracked, petulant individual. I could feel the deep wounds her senseless rages inflicted on my father, myself and the younger children. It was this frightful experience that later directed my interest as a physician to the problem of the menopause.

We know very little about this mother who so galvanised her son into making his personal life political, but we can picture her easily enough. Her son's book came out only three years after the American feminist Betty Friedan lifted the shrouds from 'The Feminine Mystique' in her book of the same title and challenged the notion that women should be home-bound perfect mothers, devoted solely to cooking, cleaning, the acquisition of labour-saving appliances and putting on a pretty face, frock and teetering high heels for a husband returning from the office. Mrs Wilson, one suspects, would have been less wracked by the nightmare of raising teenagers in the 1940s and 1950s if she'd gone out and got herself a job or a spot of voluntary work. Her son did all right out of it, though. Not everyone agreed with his extreme view, but the market value of oestrogen rose dramatically in the US between 1963 and 1973 and Dr Wilson's medical practice was a rip-roaring success.

Wendy Cooper, a British journalist working on the London *Evening News*, became interested in HRT in 1973 when she was researching a series of articles which she called 'A Change for the Better'. The articles became a book called *No Change*, which was first published in 1975 and in which she says, 'Just once or twice in the life of a working journalist comes a story so exciting, important and demanding that it refuses to be written out or written off.' For her that story was HRT. She researched her subject in Britain and the United States and *No Change* was the first analysis of this revolutionary new treatment written for women by a woman.

Cooper was 51 and took HRT herself, which reinforced her faith in it. I should say at this juncture that my own mother was in the throes of menopausal symptoms at the time of publication and was threatened with a hysterectomy. I was sent a copy of *No Change* prior to interviewing Wendy Cooper and was so impressed by her theory that menopause had been seen for too long as a natural and inevitable process that women must suffer and be neglected or dismissed as hysterical by the medical profession, that I sent my mother a copy too. Her GP was open-minded enough to agree to have a go and she took HRT for more than 20 years, into her seventies. She saved herself from the surgeon's knife and looked and felt quite marvellous.

Cooper hails Wilson as the man at the forefront of what she saw as a biological revolution to make the menopause obsolete and she excused his worst excesses:

> *Dr Wilson felt that the new discoveries should be changing these laissez-faire medical attitudes. He set out quite deliberately to shock what he called the 'Nice-Nellies' of either sex, many of them doctors, by describing the menopausal women as castrates deprived of sexual function. And he went on to draw a horrifying picture of the post-menopausal woman, liable to drying tissues, weakening muscles, sagging skin, brittle bones and shrinking vagina. If there was an element of overstatement in this, at least as shock tactics it worked.*

Wendy Cooper saw herself writing as a woman for women in the age of Women's Lib and describes her approach as more rational than romantic, with less emphasis on femininity than feminism. In this context she defines feminism as the right of women to have more say in decisions, whether they be medical or social, which affect their own lives. She acknowledged that, while admiring Wilson for pushing the issue into the public arena, he was to be recognised as a man driven by the popular prejudices of his gender:

> *Dr Wilson's book was based strongly, not only on his convictions and attitudes as a doctor, but on his convictions and attitudes as a man, betraying a romantic regard that amounts to reverence for the mysterious core of womanhood which he calls femininity. This quality, a subtle blend of the sexual and emotional rooted deep in our correct hormone balance, could be, he believes, cruelly extinguished by what he terms the castrating effects of the menopause, leaving a neutered, devalued creature, deserving man's pity rather than his passion.*

Cooper ended her book with a manifesto for a future which failed to foresee the reluctance of a number of women, young and old, to ingest a daily medicine, be it the contraceptive pill or HRT:

> I believe the young women of today, used to their daily hormone contraceptive pill will find that, by the time they reach the menopause, it will be equally accepted for them to be given the lower dosage of hormones that will eliminate the problem failing ovaries can bring. It will be as natural to combat these aspects of ageing as it is now to have eyes tested and to be given a prescription for the right lenses. Replacing hormone deficiency at the menopause will be as automatic as it is now to replace thyroid deficiency or use insulin. And, maybe, when the words Women's Lib are no more than the remembered echo of some old battle cry from an ancient victory, the words 'biological lib' will continue to have meaning for women as the basic freedom, designed not to decry the female role, but to control and maintain it.

By the early 1970s in the US half of all women aged 55 to 64 and a third aged 65 to 74 were taking oestrogen. Premarin – the first branded HRT – had become one of the top five best-selling drugs in the States. Meanwhile, in the UK during the first half of the 1970s prescriptions for hormonal preparations had been rising steadily, reaching a peak between 1976 and 1977. Prescription figures went up from 500,000 in 1972 to 1.3 million in 1976, but still only 3 per cent of the target age were getting HRT. The press was just beginning to highlight the greater availability in both countries with newspaper articles, TV programmes and, of course, Wendy Cooper's book.

Cooper was at the forefront of those feminists who embraced HRT and berated those doctors who were reluctant, as Gail Vines, the award-winning science journalist and author of *Raging Hormones*, puts it, to show anything other than indifference to women's health and who were keen to label their female patients neurotic. It's a view shared by Jo Wagerman, the first woman to become chairman of the British Board of Jewish Deputies and an HRT taker since her menopause at the age of 52. She's now 67. She is not a woman to be fobbed off or messed with, but she and many of her friends have found the attitudes of most male doctors 'forbidding'.

A great many of them, she thinks, consider it nonsense that women should want HRT and see it as evidence of their foolishness in seeking eternal youth. She sees reluctance to prescribe as an important gender issue and feels that her experience shows a degree of resentment among some males in the profession towards women having the ability to arrest, or at least slow down, some of the worst aspects of the ageing process (her concern, you may recall, was a family history of severe osteoporosis). Also, as a woman in public life, she's suspicious. Could distaste for a preparation which is said to give women energy during their most confident and assertive time of life simply be another example of the male backlash against women taking their place in society? This dismissive attitude was not, she observes wryly, their response to Viagra, which was broadly given an excited welcome and, unlike HRT, isn't even, she says, of potential benefit to the whole male body, just one little part.

Nevertheless, the issue of HRT has seen the drawing of battle lines within the feminist camp. In *Raging Hormones* Gail Vines says that in general American feminists have been suspicious of HRT whilst on the whole their British sisters in the 1970s and 1980s were more welcoming. An academic study carried out in 1984 concluded that women in both countries had endeavoured to counteract the perceived stigma of the menopause and to highlight the difficulties of operating in both cultures as an older woman. In the US, though, the focus was to neutralise the stigma by claiming menopause is normal and not a disease. In Britain, the thrust of the argument was the claim that menopausal problems are real and not a mere figment of the imagination. The strongest female voices in Britain called for the medical profession to improve and perfect treatment and make HRT widely available to those women who choose it.

In 1975, when *No Change* was first published, Wendy Cooper had stated that Robert Wilson's primary aim was the conversion of the rest of the medical profession to HRT. The majority of gynaecologists in the US quickly became advocates, although some had reservations about long-term use and at family-doctor level there was still a great deal of ignorance. A similar situation pertained in the UK – and, frankly, still does. But in the very year Cooper was published came fuel for the anti-HRT camp. A series of articles appeared in the *New England Journal of Medicine* linking ERT – we say tomarto, they say tomayto, we spell it oestrogen, they spell it estrogen; another example of two nations divided by the same language – to increased rates of endometrial cancer, which is a malignancy in the lining of the womb. It was suggested there was up to a seven-fold risk. The scare was widely reported and had an immediate and enormous impact. The demand for prescriptions plummeted and there was heated debate throughout the medical community. The researchers Harry Ziel and William Finkle observed:

> The endocrinologist who gives estrogen as treatment for the menopause is hoping to prevent senescence. His patient is readily deluded by her wish to preserve her figure and by her physician's implication that estrogen promises eternal youth. In a rational approach to therapy, risk is weighed against benefit.

In 1976, a leader in the *British Medical Journal* urged caution in the use of oestrogen in the light of the US findings. By 1980 it was widely accepted that the increased risk of endometrial cancer in

HRT-takers, compared with women who had never taken HRT, was three to six times greater. It was at this point that it was realised that giving women oestrogen, unopposed by progesterone – the hormone which balances out the stimulation of the lining of the womb – was misguided. These findings led to the standard addition of progesterone, usually in its synthetic form, known as progestogen, to HRT for all women, apart from those who have had a hysterectomy and consequently have no concerns about the lining of the womb. Oestrogen, used in combination with progesterone, is known as combined or opposed therapy.

As a result of the endometrial cancer scare the hormone bubble burst and the debate intensified among the medical profession, the press and the public. There was another dramatic fall in prescriptions for HRT in both the UK and the US. There was further evidence of the mounting controversy when, in March 1975, the drug company Schering was widely criticised for a launching a new preparation, Progynova, without first informing the medical profession and in 1976 a leader in the medical journal, the *Lancet*, fired a broadside across the bows of the industry as a whole: 'The prospect of universal treatment of a large section of the female population is clearly a glittering prize for the pharmaceutical manufacturer.'

Feminists and women's groups had taken an interest in the health issues from the beginning. In 1969, Barbara Seaman (how many times must she have had to spell out her name to fend off the obvious jokes?) published *The Doctors' Case Against the Pill*. She led the campaign to force the Nelson hearings on the safety of the pill carried out in the US, to take evidence from women. Then, in 1977, she published a critical work on ERT, *Women and the crisis in sex hormones*, which followed a year after the famous feminist text *Our Bodies, Ourselves* by the Boston Women's Health Collective. Also in 1977 came another book, Rosetta Reitz's *Menopause: A Positive Approach*. All these American feminists questioned the medicalisation of the menopause and took seriously those women who reported unpleasant side-effects of hormone medication.

It was lobbying from women's groups in the US such as the National Women's Health Network which encouraged the Federal Drugs Administration (FDA) to issue an order requiring that a warning note of potential side effects should be placed in every packet of oestrogen from 1977. The drug companies were not happy. Direct opposition to the FDA's plan came from them and from the American Pharmaceutical Manufacturers' Association. Their action argued that patient information would reduce the sales of oestrogen products and therefore profits. They lost, but were backed by the American College of Obstetricians and Gynaecologists, which maintained that giving information to patients violated doctors' rights. It was up to them, they argued, to decide how much information they should disclose to patients. The FDA's position, they said, threatened the autonomy of the medical profession.

Thus, HRT and the oestrogen controversy of the 1970s began to turn aside the old-fashioned belief that doctors were all-knowing gods and to introduce the concepts of patient power and informed consent which form the basis of correct medical practice in the new century. Sandra Coney, a New Zealand journalist who published *The menopause industry* in the UK in 1995, says:

> *The news that an apparently beneficial drug, given to well women, could cause cancer, led to the troubling idea in women's minds that doctors could not necessarily be trusted. They had been duped, lulled into a false sense of the promise of professional competence. Doctors may have been duped too, but this didn't alter the fact that they had been given the reassurance that the therapy was safe. It seemed that women would have to be more alert and reject blind dependence on the medical profession. There was increasing talk about the need to involve women in decision-making about their health, especially well women.*

HRT was to some degree rehabilitated during the 1980s when its use as a long-term preventive measure, rather than a short-term reliever of symptoms such as hot flushes, began to be researched and publicised. Its potential for preventing diseases such as osteoporosis and coronary heart disease made it seem a more attractive option to those women who thought themselves at risk. The medical profession, too, became more ready to accept a treatment that could be seen to have both long- and short-term beneficial effects.

The arguments, however, have not abated and with each generation has come a new 'menopause manifesto' for or against hormone replacement therapy. Wendy Cooper typified the side which has continued to argue that, at last, women can be liberated from a condition which for too long was dismissed as part of the natural ageing process or was simply 'all in the mind'. Commentators such as Cooper still contend, as we saw in Jo Wagerman's comments, that the medical establishment's slowness to take up HRT can be interpreted as doctors' indifference to women's health and their keenness to label women as neurotic.

Dr Marion Everitt runs one of only four National Health Service self-referral menopause clinics in Britain. Hers is in Leeds. As a woman who has reached seniority in her profession and chosen to practise in the field of women's health, she represents a relatively new trend in medicine. Marion told me she has no qualms about treating menopause as a deficiency disease. With diabetes or a malfunction of the thyroid, she says, we would have no worries about prescribing the appropriate medication, insulin or thyroxin, which we would then expect the patient to take for the rest of his or her life. She sees no difference with regard to the menopause. There is, in her view, a clear and measurable deficiency which can be boosted to beneficial effect and, she challenges, why not?

The other side, as we've seen, objects to the medicalisation of the menopause as a deficiency disease and the creation of a menopause industry. This fits in with a wider theme of second-wave feminism which has consistently tried to place value on women's own definitions and experiences rather than placing blind and respectful faith in those of the medical profession. This approach has served to give women greater influence, not only in managing their own menopause, but in the fields of pregnancy and childbirth too. Those who belong to the anti-HRT camp have also argued that doctors such as Robert Wilson have frightened women into seeking out the medical approach because of an exaggerated portrayal of the 'inevitable' miseries of an ugly, decrepit and deficient old age and the social pressure to continue to be a 'girl' woman – slender, fit, wrinkle-free and sexually attractive to men.

The most vociferous foot soldier for this camp is Germaine Greer, whose book, *The Change*, was first published in 1991, is a searing attack on a society which has ignored or derided its middle-aged women for centuries, noticing them only when there's a chance to dope them up to fit into the cult of youth and make a bunch of money out of their hunger for relief of their menopausal symptoms. At the same time, she welcomes the opportunity for personal development that the menopause offers. It's a chance, she argues, to embrace our non-reproductive selves and become again the people we were before we became 'tools' of our sexual and reproductive systems. We need, in her view, to devise new rites of passage for ourselves, in order to celebrate what could be regarded as the restoration of the woman to herself, free from demanding children, needy men and elderly relatives.

Greer is critical of the medical profession for arresting this natural process artificially by prescribing HRT, which she believes has been dished out like sweets without enough testing. The consequence of the race to relieve symptoms – the main thrust of the industry – has led us to ignore any opportunity to research those women who do not have unpleasant experiences during menopause and to find out why some women do not suffer whilst others do.

The silver lining to what can be a very dark cloud during this time is, she thinks, a liberation from passion and the chance to enter contented celibacy. She sees life without sex as truly freeing women from the onerous responsibilities which are often a social consequence of their relationships with men. The post-menopausal woman has, she says, the chance to be independently powerful. She advises the reclamation of the words 'witch' and 'crone' and says, 'You're expected to be dreadful, so why not act it?' Most of us, I suspect, like Melba Wilson, are happy to become more assertive in middle age, but aren't yet ready to chuck the old man out!

Greer's thesis didn't go down well with me and she had a number of other detractors. Some commentators accused her of taking women back in time, with her talk of witches, crones and hags. My view is that reclamation is one thing, making ourselves a hostage to already outrageous fortune is quite another – do we really need to encourage our sons to address us as old hags? I think not. Then, of course, whilst Germaine is always the most provocative of all our thinkers, it's difficult to pity a woman with a razor-sharp intellect and cheekbones to match. Her manifesto for celibacy with its call for us to revel in a lack of sexual allure has a hollow ring, coming from a woman who'll be 'drop-dead gorgeous' in her coffin.

Gail Sheehy, the American author of *The Silent Passage*, published in the UK in 1993, takes issue with Germaine Greer's school of thought. What is lost for Sheehy in the arguments between the 'menopause as a disease' group and the proponents of 'menopause as a natural event' is what she sees as the main point: 'that we are living longer lives than ever before. Since there has been virtually no period in the history of the human species when evolution has favoured post-menopausal females, we shall have to favour ourselves. We shall have to intervene, medically, hormonally, psychologically, spiritually – because we cannot assume that ageing will go smoothly.'

Sheehy's aim, like mine, is to break the taboo surrounding the menopause, which, almost ten years after the publication of her book, patently still exists. In her conclusion, she calls for women to enter a new state of post-menopausal equilibrium: 'Think of it as discarding the shell of the reproductive self – who came into being in adolescence – and coming out the other side to coalescence.' (*Author's note*: the dictionary definition of 'coalesce' is to unite or come together in one body or mass; merge; fuse; blend – if that's helpful!)

Sandra Coney, author of *The Menopause Industry* (1995), opens her treatise thus: 'If the world was kinder to women, this book need never have been written.' Like Greer, she argues that women in mid-life are well, but are conditioned to be preoccupied with disease. She rails against a medical profession that has 'discovered' the mid-life woman and made her disease into a profit-making industry and says, 'Medicine depoliticises the situation of the mid-life woman by reducing her socially caused anxieties and complaints to symptoms of bodily processes that can be solved by medication.' Women, she claims, then get sucked into the medical traps of the menopause industry.

She is also critical, however, of the happy-clappy feminist view which calls for a redefinition of the menopause as entirely positive. This is, she argues, too idealistic and excludes women who do encounter difficulties: 'Feminist ideology runs the risk of denying women's actual experience. The effect can be that women blame themselves for not coping better.'

Coney also introduces the idea of social and cultural influences on the way women perceive their middle years and indeed their old age (does anybody ever get called old any more – and if not why not? See Chapter 8). She claims that 'Whether menopause is seen as a negative, positive or neutral event will depend on factors such as social attitudes to older women and the status accorded women's reproductive role. In defining menopause for herself, the individual woman will draw on the current stereotype of menopause in her own culture.'

There is some evidence to demonstrate that this is true and it does offer a powerful counter-argument to the belief that menopause is a disease. Melba Wilson, who is black, did suffer from heavy periods, night sweats and hot flushes, which were a profound irritation during meetings, especially as she had just taken on a high-powered new job as the policy director of the mental health charity, MIND. But black women, she says, age differently from white ones. She expresses her belief with caution, only too aware of the stereotypes that can surround the black woman; she's either an aggressive matriarch who can cope with anything life throws at her or an oversexed hot mama, carrying from slavery the legacy of the misguided belief that a black woman is ever ready and always available.

She did observe, though, that all her white friends were rushing for HRT and not discussing too much what was happening to them, whereas she discussed it with her mother when she came close to following their lead. Her mother told her she had had similar symptoms, had just 'toughed it out' and was then fine. Her friend, Bel Gilroy, now in her seventies, described her village in Guyana, where the women would make themselves a 'tea potion' and talk about their physical symptoms. Menopause was treated as a rite of passage and the women helped each other to get through it.

Melba also says that all the women she is close to have felt their bodies were beautiful. They have acknowledged that, because they are black, they are not considered attractive to society at large – the thin white woman has always been considered the ideal, so black women have been free to accept themselves collectively for what they are. The older black woman is, she says, revered and respected within her own society, so there are plenty of role models. Both males and females are considered attractive if they are well covered. Big bottoms are in! So, now that her body is beginning to look like her mother's, she appreciates, rather than fears it.

Angela Mason is now 55 and has run Stonewall, the organisation which works for equality for gay men and lesbians, since her late forties. She too took on a big job as she became menopausal. Her consciousness of her body is, she says, almost zero. She recalls heavy periods for a year or two – which she remembers causing her real problems only once. It was her first Labour Party Conference as director and Tony Blair's first as leader and she had to rush off to the loo in Brighton just before introducing him at their fringe meeting to pre-empt the possibility of flooding. Apart from that, she had no real anxieties, but went to her doctor for HRT almost as a matter of course, to fix her hot sweats.

Angela knows nothing about HRT and asked no questions, but will take it for as long as she's told. She has, she says, no real relationship with her body's functions, which she puts down in part to her sexuality. Heterosexual women, she explains, are more conscious of their periods because each time they have sex they might get pregnant. This is not the case for lesbians, except for a short while if they choose to become parents. For Angela and her partner of many years, Elizabeth, it was only for the short period, when Angela was trying to conceive their now teenage daughter, Ellie.

Nor, she says, has she ever had to play the sex card in mixed company. Flirting to advance her career was never an option, so her experience of her sexual identity has been constant thoughout her life and hasn't changed with age. As for Melba, spending a lot of time in the company of women has meant she has had role models – women who have gone through the difficult bits, to emerge confident and well on the other side. Elizabeth went through it all before her. Angela believes that in the lesbian community people of different ages generally mix together, so the cult of youth is less of a pressure on the old. Consequently, she thinks, her menopause and beyond has been a minor inconvenience rather than a major trauma.

The literature on culture is brimming with other examples. In *Raging Hormones*, Gail Vines writes:

> one school of thought promoted particularly by feminist primatologists and anthropologists begins with the 'grandmother hypothesis'. In this view, menopause has evolved because it maximises the reproductive output of the woman and her close kin. Through her labour and experience, the post-menopausal grandmother contributes to the survival of her children and their children.

She quotes evidence in favour of this idea from a study of the Hadza hunter gatherers in Tanzania:

> Post-reproductive Hadza women specialise in collecting tubers which are a nutrituous and valuable source of food, but difficult to dig up. Younger women with children do not have time to harvest them. The older women spend more time gathering food and bring in more than their younger relatives. So, through their skilled labour, the older women greatly enhance their kin's food supply. Menopause is not, then, a disease or a debilitating state, but a valued stage in human life which first arose because it carried evolutionary advantages.

Another theory argues the menopause is Nature's original contraceptive that freed women for leadership in the extended family and the community:

In pre-capitalist or pre-literate societies, pregnancy and childbirth themselves are dangerous; survival is anything but assured. The woman who finally makes it and finds herself assuming authority over new daughters-in-law and running the large household, must usually have done so during the climacterum [echoes of Shirley William's view of Margaret Thatcher here], but we would be surprised to find any significant amount of evidence relating to its discomforts on the part of women who have everything to congratulate themselves upon having reached it.

This sense of triumph was echoed by Melba Wilson, who told me that a number of her friends had died in their forties from breast or liver cancer, so she considered getting to 50 a privilege.

It was also Melba, you'll recall – perhaps the most confident of all the post-menopausal women to whom I have spoken – who talked of becoming more assertive and stronger in her personal relationships. This may no longer be so necessary for the running of a large, dependent household of children, except in the more traditional homes in the Asian community, but it may be vital in the new demographics in choosing whether or not to look after a sick and ageing parent or partner or, as Vera Ivers has done, becoming a local councillor. The journalist, Linda Grant, wrote movingly about her decision to put her mother in a nursing home, rather than give up her career as a writer in order to care for her. Her mother was suffering from a form of dementia and Linda says without the understanding of her feminist friends and the political background of the women's movement, this choice would not have been open to her. Equally, a number of older women have taken on positions in national politics in the House of Lords, alongside their own professions. Baroness Kennedy, for example, has teenage children, sits on a number of voluntary boards and decision-making bodies and still practises law as Helena Kennedy, QC. I doubt she would want to be worried about having more children as well.

We know that even in the most restricitive societies women are granted a greater degree of freedom after menopause than they were permitted in their reproductive years because they no longer represent a risk of pollution. Frequently, menstruating women are set apart from family and friends and are not allowed to touch or prepare certain foods because their menstruation is believed to taint or pollute. Even when free from menstruation, they are often kept within the household or allowed out only when fully covered, so as not to be seen as sex objects through whom their husbands might be dishonoured.

Perhaps the most famous anecdotal tale is that women in Japan don't even have a word for hot flushes or night sweats. The anthropologist Margaret Lock has researched *koneki*, the Japanese word for menopause. After interviewing numerous doctors and women and sending out questionnaires, she found that the doctors spoke of a list of symptoms connected to *koneki*, but women reported fewer, citing headaches, aching and ringing in the ears. The most commonly reported symptom was stiff shoulder, reported by 52 per cent. (One wonders whether the considerable weight of the kimono becomes more arduous with age, but Lock didn't ask the question!) Hot flush was mentioned by only 10 per cent and night sweats by 3 per cent and, indeed, the language does not have an accepted word for them. Neither, interestingly, does Thai. Instead, the term *ork horn wuup waap* – heat sensation intermittently – is used. It's the same terminology as that for a burn or the feeling you get from touching a hot chilli.

Most of the women and doctors questioned said they associated *koneki* with a natural, gradual ageing process rather than hormones and felt it was represented more commonly by greying hair and failing eyesight than with the cessation of menstruation. The women who were asked if they saw themselves as menopausal rarely answered that they saw the menopause as coinciding with the end of their periods – indeed, some women who had not menstruated for more than 12 months still said they didn't have any signs of the menopause. Lock concluded that for 65 per cent of Japanese women, menopause is uneventful.

The virtual non-existence of hot flushes among Japanese women cannot be explained solely by cultural attitudes, but by physical factors too. Their diet is higher in phyto-oestrogens than the Western diet, and this has also been linked to their lower rates of breast cancer and osteoporosis. (There'll be more on this subject in Chapter 7.) It would be interesting to return to Japan some years hence and find whether creeping Westernisation has influenced women and their menopause. Lock found that the Japanese press has recently begun to talk of 'menopausal syndrome' – describing it as a disease of modernity and a luxury disease, affecting women with too much time on their hands who run to their doctors with insignificant complaints. Japanese gynaecologists working in private clinics have begun to promote HRT.

Recent research among Thai women found that only 23 per cent suffered from hot flushes and 17 per cent listed sweating as a problem. Headaches and dizziness were associated with the menopause, but forgetfulness and sleeplessness were seen as normal age-related complaints. Emotional problems or depression were linked to economic and personal circumstances, not to changes in the menstrual cycle.

Another anthropologist, Marcha Flint, believes that 'whether menopause is viewed as reward or punishment may be critical to women's experience'. From her studies of women in the Rajput caste of northern India, she found that the end of menstruation was liberating because a woman was allowed to emerge from purdah and was free for the first time since girlhood to socialise freely in her community. Women looked forward to the menopause and had virtually no symptoms.

Similar attitudes were found amongst women in Mayan villages. When one study asked them about hot flushes, the researchers drew blank stares, while women of a similar racial and cultural background who now live in cities said they did experience them, suggesting they are picking up on the attitudes of their adopted culture. There are some suggestions that these differences may be explained biologically. Direct comparisons are troublesome when cultures vary so starkly in their patterns of childbearing and their attitudes to the pregnant woman or new mother. It could be that hot flushes are less meaningful in hotter climates where a sudden bout of sweating would have less of an impact on the individual or those around them.

The most recently published evidence comes from Gabriella Berger who, in her book *Menopause and Culture*, compares the experiences of Australian and Filipino women. Her studies showed that, as in other Western countries, up to 80 per cent of Australian women suffer from moderate to severe menopausal symptoms, while for Filipino women it's around 40 per cent. Berger explored a number of cultural factors and concluded that cultural expectations of menopause are most probably a self-fulfilling prophecy. For example, Filipino women are culturally expected to feel irritable, so they say they do. Women who had less information about what was expected of them at menopause were unsure of their symptoms. Australian women had more difficulty coming to terms with ageing than did the Filipino women, who mentioned that they received more respect and had a strong grandmother role. On the positive side for the Australian women was what they saw as a licence to worry less about what people thought of them.

Teresa Gorman tells me of an anthropological study of the 'Blue' people of Morocco which she heard described at a conference on the menopause some years ago. In this tribe girls at puberty are given a sash which they must wear at all times to signify their fertility. When they reach menopause they are expected to abandon it and wear only black to denote their new status as doyenne of the family, a grandmotherly figure. Apparently, they cheat, knowing that if they do choose to drop the sash their husband will be given carte blanche to go off with a younger woman – and they're not having that! Teresa's theory is that the whole idea of the older woman as head of the household is just another myth sustained by people who want women kept in their place rather than taking an active role in the community. These Moroccan women, she reckons, have worked out their own way of achieving what's best for them. Effectively keeping themselves out of the mental hospital and out of the divorce court!

With all the widely divergent cultural attitudes and feminist perceptions of what the menopause signifies and, indeed, whether or not it is a treatable disease at all, it's hardly suprising that the battleground currently extends to the medical profession itself. I began the chapter with a friend's irritation at a doctor's glib definition of the deficiencies caused by a condition he believes we were never meant to have, while Dr Marion Everitt is clear in her conviction that menopause is a deficiency disease and has no hesitation about prescribing. Lots of women told me they weren't interested in HRT, but the doctor mentioned it every time they went to the surgery. Other doctors, as Jo Wagerman found, are reluctant to listen to women or to prescribe. Disagreements are not only about medical evidence, but the way people, including doctors, view the menopause. So when can you rely on the old saying, Trust me, I'm a doctor?

CHAPTER 3

TRUST ME, I'M A DOCTOR

Edwina Currie, a former minister for health and now a best-selling novelist of 54, describes the start of her menopause when she was 48 as:

> walking into a brick wall. I was lethargic, frightened, tense and anxious, which is not like me at all. I began to bleed heavily and more frequently, so I kept notes of the new menstrual pattern for a few months and took the diary to a doctor. He was keen and modern, so it was a bit of a shock when his first words to me after I'd described my problem were, 'The waiting list for a hysterectomy is only four months!'

I have to say, my jaw had to be picked up from the floor when Edwina told me this story. If she could be treated like this, I wondered, what hope is there for those of us who don't have her vast experience of the health service or, to put it bluntly, her ability to argue on her own behalf?

Even Edwina, not known for her reticence, was temporarily silenced and when she did finally speak it was to ask, in strangled tones, whether he thought she had cancer. It's bizarre, but even the feistiest among us are reduced to asking stupid questions when the medical profession puts the fear of God into us. The doctor's response was to talk for 20 minutes about how easy hysterectomies are to perform these days which, happily, gave her time to think. Yes, she'd had fibroids (non-cancerous tumours) in the past, as have lots of women, and, like most of us, she'd suffered no significant trouble. It was obviously insensitive of him to suggest a hysterectomy without first making further investigations. At the very least he should have offered a blood test to assess hormone levels and decide whether the new bleeding pattern was simply a result of the menopause or whether the fibroids were beginning to be bothersome.

Edwina walked out of the surgery, with a 'fine, I'll go away and think.' She immediately called an old gynaecologist friend. His was a less radical, but somewhat unorthodox response. Nevertheless it suited Edwina. He gave her some tablets, told her to take them and said, 'If you don't feel better by the time you get home, we're on the wrong track.'

She swallowed the pills, oestrogen – as it turned out – drove to Derby, called him and told him she felt a lot better. She spent the next year or so going back and forth, checking what level of replacement her system needed (as we'll show in Chapters 4 and 5, it can take some time to get it right) but she avoided an operation and carried on with her rudely healthy lifestyle. Which, of course, is the way most of us should feel in our middle years. We should all expect to be as well as we've always been, full of beans and enthusiasm for whatever we've chosen to do. A minority of women will experience some form of ill health at this stage of life, but most of us are fit as fleas.

Here are the facts about health risks affecting us in the middle years. Death rates at all ages above 45 are lower in women than men. We live, on average, five years longer, but see our doctors more often – a result, no doubt, of getting into the habit whilst we sought contraception, had our babies and then took them to the surgery for childhood illnesses and vaccinations. The higher attendance rate has led to a false assumption that women are sicker than men. Not so.

Overall, coronary heart disease is the biggest single cause of death in women, exceeded slightly by all the different cancers combined. The older we get, the more likely we are to die from diseases of the circulatory system than from cancer. The major causes of disability from 45 to 105 are disorders of the bones and joints. Some of us will have higher or lower risk factors depending on our genes, family history, lifestyle and whether or not we have a premature menopause.

It's an important cautionary tale Edwina Currie tells and emphasises how informed we need to be and how ready to stand up for what we want when going to a doctor's surgery. Not all of us can choose our doctors or have friends in high places to whom we can run for advice if the system seems to be failing us. Most of us are stuck with a doctor, although on p. 283 you will find a list of organisations that can be phoned for extra information if you need someone to talk to after reading this book. The crucial thing to remember is not to get scared and not to be bamboozled into anything you're not sure about. It's an old piece of advice, but it does help to write down your questions and feelings on a piece of paper before you go to a doctor, otherwise even the best informed and connected among us can become tongue-tied. If you are unhappy with the doctor's assessment, ask to see someone in the practice who specialises in women of this age group. If that fails, try one of the few self-referral clinics (see Useful Addresses). If it can happen to Edwina Currie it can happen to any of us!

The story does, perhaps, give some idea as to why a recent MORI poll found that 75 per cent of 45- to 65-year-old women complained of unpleasant and uncomfortable menopausal symptoms ranging from hot flushes to depression, but 3 in 10 of those women had not consulted a doctor. Some of us will simply be stoical, determined to weather the menopause as our mothers and grandmothers did. Some of us may be afraid that we'll be pushed into taking treatments which may not be safe in the long term. Both these approaches are fine, so long as the peri-menopausal symptoms are no more serious than those we've already discussed: periods becoming a little heavier or lighter or stopping altogether.

The next section is intended to pick out those occasions when you may need to see a doctor, examine how you feel about screening and give some idea of how to make decisions about treatment if you do become one of the few who need it. (Before going any further, if you are having menopausal symptoms you may find it worthwhile having your thyroid checked out. Many complications of low thyroid function can be confused with the symptoms of the menopause, and include osteoporosis, high cholesterol, tiredness, weight gain, constipation, dry skin, brittle hair and menstrual irregularities. Your doctor can easily check this with a blood test.)

BLEEDING PROBLEMS

It is advisable to consult a doctor if you have stopped menstruating for more than a year and then start again; if you experience flooding on a regular basis; if you have bleeding in between periods; if you have bleeding accompanied by severe pain and a high temperature; or if you bleed after sex.

Apart from the menopause, this abnormal bleeding, with or without pain, could be caused by a number of factors, including problems with an intra-uterine device (contraceptive coil), gynaecological cancers, endometrial hyperplasia (overgrowth of the uterine lining), endometriosis (a chronic condition where the cells which form the lining of the womb develop outside their normal location); fibroids (lumps of fibrous and muscular tissue growing on the walls of the uterus); polyps in the cervix or uterine lining; ovarian cysts; pelvic inflammatory disease, known as PID (an infection in the uterus or the Fallopian tubes); ectopic pregnancy or miscarriage.

SELF-HELP

- Keep a menstrual diary – it will be helpful when you go for a consultation.
- If you have what you consider to be heavy periods (and this can be a subjective assessment for every woman, depending on what her normal cycle has been like) it is worth taking extra iron and B-group vitamins with vitamin C to offset the danger of becoming anaemic.

MEDICAL HELP

If menstrual irregularities are the result of the menopause and nothing more serious (and this can only be established by testing – not, as we've seen, by those doctors who see hysterectomy as the panacea for all ills 'down below') and you are not keen to try HRT, there are drugs – mefenamic acid (Ponstan) and tranexamic acid (Cyclokapron) – which can reduce heavy bleeding. Professor Angela Coulter, director of the King's Fund Centre in London, has said that 'a lot of women are going on to have unnecessary hysterectomies because they are not being offered better drug treatment.'

Hormone treatment is another option. Progestogen can balance out excessive build-up of the lining of the womb in response to oestrogen. It can be administered in the form of a tablet or a Mirena – a slow-release coil, similar to that used in contraception, which can be inserted into the uterus. This was Rosie Thomas's choice after she experienced her severe haemorrhaging whilst in the Himalayas. It is currently licensed in this country as a treatment for heavy bleeding, but not yet as a hormone replacement therapy. Dr Marion Everitt of the Leeds Menopause Clinic tells me that where a Mirena has been used in hospitals as a treatment for heavy bleeding, the rate of hysterectomy has been halved. She describes it as the best thing for women's health since the pill. (More on this in Chapter 4.) The most commonly prescribed drug, Norethisterone, which is a progesterone hormone, has been found to be no more effective than a placebo at the doses normally prescribed.

HRT may be suggested to treat irregular bleeding and possibly reduce heavy bleeding.

HYSTERECTOMY

Nearly 100,000 hysterectomies are carried out each year. Data published in October 2000, showing the first results from the Million Women Study into the health of British women aged 50 to 64 and funded by the NHS and leading medical researchers, says 1 in 4 women in the study has had her womb removed. Only in the United States is the figure higher: 1 in 3. This is possibly the result of American doctors practising a more defensive type of medicine, given the litigious nature of the country. More cynically, a system of private medicine may tempt surgeons to operate when it is not really necessary. In Scandinavia, scarcely 1 woman in 10 has had the operation by the time she retires and in France the rate is half that of the UK. French women and their doctors regard the womb as a vital organ to be preserved if possible and if large fibroids give trouble, doctors will remove the fibroids rather than the uterus. They are willing to give repeat operations for large fibroids if necessary although there can be more post-operative complications than with hysterectomy.

In Britain, in at least half the cases, menorrhagia (heavy bleeding) is the main complaint and, in half of those cases, the uterus turns out to be completely normal. The number of hysterectomies performed varies in different parts of the country. This could be due to the social conditions in which the patients live or it could vary depending on the different attitudes of surgeons in the different regions.

The hysterectomy rate increased dramatically in this country from the 1950s to the 1980s and it is now one of the most commonly performed operations in Britain. In February 2000 the Royal College of Obstetricians and Gynaecologists was worried enough about numbers and regional variations to launch new guidelines for doctors on managing menorrhagia. The guidelines asked doctors to examine their own practise in the light of the variations that have been shown to exist in the level of investigating carried out before surgery, treatment with drugs and operative procedures. There was a course to examine the issues involving some of the leading consultants in the field.

At the end of July 1999, the private health insurance company BUPA had introduced measures which required consultant gynaecologists to get prior authorisation before going ahead with a hysterectomy under the private system. Where heavy bleeding is the only symptom, BUPA will pay for the operation only after three months of alternative treatments have been tried. BUPA had been alarmed by surveys which showed that of all the hysterectomies carried out in the UK each year, up to 25 per cent may have been unnecessary.

The move angered the British Medical Association, which accused BUPA of unwarranted interference in clinical decisions. From our point of view as consumers there are, of course, powerful vested interests to be considered here. BUPA want to pay only for cost-effective, appropriate treatment, and doctors want to be seen as independent in deciding what is best for the patient. It's helpful to know the figures involved. BUPA paid for 3600 hysterectomies at an average cost of £3890. Of that sum,

the consultant performing the operation received an average of
£790. When you consider a surgeon might perform several
hysterectomies in the course of a morning – the disgraced Kent
gynaecologist, Rodney Ledward, who styled himself the fastest
scalpel in the Southeast, boasted seven completed between 8am
and 12 noon – that's a tidy five-and-a-half grand for a morning's
work. A nice little earner.

A hysterectomy may have to be performed in cases of:
• cancer or suspected cancer of the uterus. Traditionally, gynaecologists have defended carrying out hysterectomies together
  with oophorectomy because removing the womb and ovaries
  will take away the risk of ovarian cancer, but ovarian cancer
  is rare – 3–4000 cases a year in the UK female population of
  28 million (of which ¾'s are diagnosed late)
• prolapsed uterus or vagina (where the womb has dropped some
  years after childbirth)
• pelvic inflammatory disease which is painful enough to interfere
  with daily activities
• endometriosis which has failed to respond to all other treatments and is painful enough to interfere with daily activities
• fibroids (non-cancerous tumours of the uterus) that are causing
  heavy periods and have not responded to medical treatment.
  (Other forms of treatment are now also available – see below.)
• large or multiple ovarian cysts

A hysterectomy is unlikely to be the best option for:
• endometriosis with minor symptoms
• small fibroids that cause little trouble
• general symptoms of the menopause
(However, the latter two reasons are the most common and
account for half the hysterectomies performed annually.)

Types of hysterectomy
- Sub-total – removal of the uterus, leaving the cervix in place
- Total – removal of the uterus and cervix
- Total hysterectomy with oophorectomy/bilateral oophorectomy – includes the removal of one or both ovaries
- Radical – removal of the uterus, part of the vagina, the Fallopian tubes and ovaries
  (Note: When the uterus and ovaries are removed, a woman will generally receive HRT to treat premature menopause. The operation can be performed via an incision in the stomach or through the vagina. Recovery is quicker and the complications minimised with the latter. It is only useful for treating women who have a hysterectomy to deal with heavy periods and it is among this group that the operation is least likely to be necessary.)

Risks
- It has a 2 per cent complication rate.
- The risk of depression is increased.
- The risk of loss of bone density and osteoporosis is increased, as is that of heart disease and urinary incontinence if the ovaries are removed without HRT being offered.

After-effects
Around 85 per cent of women who have a hysterectomy say they are satisfied with the operation. Most studies show that sex improves after the op, probably because the pain and inconvenience of heavy periods is removed. You may also remember from Chapter 1, Vera Ivers' comment that sexual desire is in the head, not the uterus. It has been found that, if it is possible for medical reasons, it is better to leave the cervix in place.

Sandra Chalmers, director of communications for Help the Aged and chairman of the Board of Trustees for the Pennell Initiative for

Women's Health, was Editor of *Woman's Hour* when, in her mid-forties, she began to have 'tremendously heavy periods. I became anaemic and terribly tired.'

A D & C had no effect, so she was advised to have a hysterectomy. She is, she confesses, very bad at asking questions and now regrets agreeing to have half an ovary left behind. She vaguely remembers being told it would allow her to have 'a natural menopause', which, in retrospect, she wishes she'd never had, as it was horrid. She had hot flushes for a long time, which were embarrassing professionally, as was her lack of concentration. Whether she regrets the hysterectomy or not is difficult to assess, as she was so relieved at the time not to have the debilitating heavy bleeding any more.

Dissatisfaction is generally related to whether the operation was done for a very good reason and after full consideration by the woman of the options available. Most of the women who suffer depression after hysterectomy are those who underwent surgery because of a non-life-threatening condition. One of the leaders in the field, Professor Stephen Smith, runs a referral clinic in Cambridge for menstrual dysfunction. He says, 'We tell women that whatever it takes, we will sort out the problem. There is a host of treatments and it is up to women to choose. Hysterectomy is only one of the options. If women were given real choice, the number of hysterectomies for heavy periods could be halved.'

Dr Susan Love, an American breast surgeon and author of *The Hormone Dilemma*, rather surprisingly, as it's her business, describes surgery as 'the ultimate breaking and entering'. She acknowledges there is a need for it at times, but she too is alarmed at the number of unnecessary operations that are carried out. Hysterectomy, she says, is often the choice with the highest risk. Not only short-term risk, but also, often, long-term consequences. 'You can stop taking a drug if it turns out to have been the wrong choice,' she advises.

'You can't put your organs back in if you find you didn't need that hysterectomy.'

Obviously, if it is suggested that you should have a hysterectomy, you need to be armed with questions and to spend time discussing the options with those responsible for your medical care. Consent forms are now much more sophisticated than they were before 1998. Point out to your doctor, if necessary, that he or she is a surgeon, not a mind-reader. You know what you want. Read through the forms carefully, discuss what you are prepared to have done once you're under anaesthetic and what not and sign accordingly.

ALTERNATIVE SURGICAL TECHNIQUES

All of these operations, although relatively new, are available on the NHS. Before agreeing to a hysterectomy, discuss these other options with your doctor. If he or she seems reluctant to consider them, see another doctor in the practice and keep trying until you get a referral to a specialist with an open mind.

- *Endometrial ablation.* There are various forms of this technique to vaporise the endometrium, including the use of a powerful laser.
- *Microwave endometrial ablation.* A new variation on the above, it's carried out under local anaesthetic and doesn't involve staying in hospital.
- *Transcervical resection of the endometrium (TCRE).* This surgical technique uses an electrically heated loop to destroy the lining of the womb down to ½ centimetre. The Royal Free Hospital in London recently carried out a study which showed that women undergoing this technique spent less time in hospital and convalesced more quickly than those who had had a hysterectomy. Some doctors feel TCRE still has to be proven and has its own risks. There is, for instance, a small risk that the uterus can be perforated during the operation.

- *Embolisation*. Cutting off the blood supply to fibroids.
- *Myomectomy (surgical removal of fibroids)*. This is still major surgery, in which each fibroid is removed and the uterus reconstructed. There are two ways of performing a myomectomy. One is to go through the cervix to the uterus if the fibroids are in the inner lining of the uterus (this is more common with the type of fibroids that cause bleeding); the other method is to enter the uterus through an incision in the abdominal wall. Keyhole surgery is possible for certain types of small fibroid.

  (If you have been taking HRT talk to your doctor about whether the oestrogen component of the treatment may have been a factor in the growth of fibroids. It may be advisable, if you choose not to have a hysterectomy, to discuss a much lower dose of oestrogen and a different form of progestogen delivery after myomectomy or to look for an alternative to HRT that will help with menopausal symptoms or long-term bone protection.)
- *Hysterectomy* is only recommended for the most severe cases of prolapse. In other cases, HRT may help to strengthen tissue structures, and in older women a PVC vaginal ring can be inserted to support the vaginal tissues. Surgery can be performed to repair the damage – and the old pelvic floor exercises, together with losing a bit of weight, can help a lot (aahh! That's what they always say, but in this case, it's true!)

CORONARY HEART DISEASE

Coronary arteries are the major blood vessels which feed the heart with its supply of oxygen. Heart disease occurs when the arteries become furred up with fatty deposits. Partial blockage of these arteries causes angina, which is characterised by pains in the chest, often after taking part in strenuous activity.

A heart attack occurs when the flow is blocked, depriving part of the heart muscle of oxygen. Nearly 20 per cent of older women who suffer heart attacks will die suddenly as a result or may find there are limitations on their daily life. Whether you survive heart attack depends on the severity of the attack and other risk factors. Women are more likely to develop angina in the first instance, which can of course be controlled with drugs, whilst men tend to have a heart attack immediately once they have developed coronary heart disease (CHD).

Men were generally thought to develop CHD some ten years before women and to die of it 20 years earlier. This difference encouraged the theory that women were protected until the menopause by their hormones. (See Chapter 5 for new research.) Some studies have also shown that women who have an early menopause, those who have their ovaries removed before the natural menopause or have a lack of hormones as a result of a number of genetic conditions, also have a higher risk of heart disease.

Researchers have found evidence that the body's own oestrogen has the ability to dilate blood vessels, helping to keep the arteries open. It also increases 'good' HDL (high-density lipoproteins) cholesterol and reduces 'bad' LDL (low-density lipoproteins) cholesterol. Twenty per cent of cholesterol comes from the food we eat and the rest is made by the body itself, mainly in the liver. In the bloodstream cholesterol is transported by the lipoproteins (combined fat and protein molecules).

High-density lipoproteins are good, because these collect cholesterol from the walls of the arteries and ferry it away again to the liver for excretion. Low-density are bad, because they carry it to fatty deposits. The ideal ratio is 3 parts HDL to 1 part LDL.

RISK FACTORS

- increasing age
- family history of heart disease
- being diabetic – diabetes increases the risk 3–7 times
- coming from a lower socio-economic group
- smoking
- being overweight – obesity doubles the likelihood of CHD
- high blood pressure
- lack of exercise
- high blood levels of cholesterol
- ethnicity – women in the UK from the Indian subcontinent are more at risk

SELF-HELP

- Have your blood pressure monitored and keep it within normal limits.
- Cut down on smoking or, better still, stop. As soon as you give up, the risk of a heart attack begins to decline and is near normal within only 3–5 years.
- Keep your weight within normal limits for your height (let's face it – we know whether we're dangerously overweight or not.)
- Take more exercise
- Have cholesterol levels checked and eat to improve good/bad ratio and reduce overall level. (More on both of these in the later diet and exercise section.)
- Drink in moderation. Moderate drinkers (one glass of wine a day) have a lower risk than heavy or non-drinkers.

You may be considering HRT to reduce your risk of CHD. It has been assumed to protect the heart by replicating the action of the body's own oestrogen. (There'll be more details of the latest research on this in Chapter 5.)

There is a word of caution in relation to heart disease and women. It has in the past been seen, typically, as a male problem. Women are only half as likely as men to be offered cardiac testing for symptoms suggesting heart problems – you may recall the tragic case of a young woman who died in the summer of 2000 in the toilets of a major London teaching hospital. She had been sent to the waiting room, presumably because staff did not immediately think 'heart attack' for a woman in her thirties. If you're worried, ask and keep on pestering.

The vast majority of studies have been carried out on men and generalised to women. So, there are many unanswered questions, such as the role and treatment of cholesterol in women, the most suitable prescriptions for blood-pressure medicines and how dietary recommendations may differ for men and women.

MEDICAL HELP

If you have a family history of heart disease, talk to your doctor about current thinking on prevention, which may include taking an aspirin a day, and have your blood pressure checked regularly.

OSTEOPOROSIS

Osteoporosis has been dubbed by the National Osteoporosis Society 'the silent epidemic', which sounds a little melodramatic, but their figures show that it affects one in three women and only one in 12 men in a lifetime. By the age of 70 a woman could have lost a third of her bone mass.

The term 'osteoporosis' means porous bones. The bones in the skeleton are made of a thick outer shell and a strong inner mesh filled with the protein collagen, calcium, salts and other minerals. The inside has the appearance of a honeycomb, with blood vessels and bone marrow in the spaces between the bone. Osteoporosis occurs when the holes between bone become bigger, making it fragile and liable to break easily. The disease usually affects the whole skeleton, but most commonly causes fractures to the wrist, spine and hip.

Bones stop growing between the ages of 16 and 18, but continue to grow in strength into the mid thirties. By this time they have reached their maximum potential strength, known as peak bone mass. Up until the age of 35 there is a balance between the breakdown of bone and its renewal, so bone density remains constant. Around the age of 40 bone loss begins to increase and renewal slows as part of the natural ageing process and in women, after the menopause, when the levels of oestrogen are dropping, the reduction of bone mass is accelerated. (There is some debate on this – see natural progesterone, p. 183.) By the age of 80, it's estimated that, without any corrective treatment, the average woman will have lost between a quarter and a half of her bone mass.

Approximately 40 per cent of all women will experience one or more fractures after the age of 50. At 80 one in five has suffered a hip fracture and at 90 it is almost one in two. Spinal fractures can cause deformity and back pain. The dowager's hump that appears in some women causes loss of height and curvature of the spine. It can also cause breathing and digestive problems. You'll remember this was Jo Wagerman's worry, as her mother and grandmother had suffered in this way and both had walked with sticks by the time they were 60.

RISK FACTORS

A lack of oestrogen caused by:
- early menopause before the age of 45
- early hysterectomy before the age of 45 (particularly if both ovaries are removed)
- missing periods for six months or more (excluding pregnancy) as a result of over-exercising or over-dieting
- anorexia

Other factors include:
- long-term use of corticosteroid tablets (for conditions such as asthma)
- maternal history of hip fracture
- inflammatory bowel disease and gastric surgery or any condition which prohibits the absorption of nutrients from food
- long-term immobility
- heavy drinking
- smoking
- low body weight
- hyperthyroidism (a very overactive thyroid left untreated)

These factors do not mean that you will inevitably suffer from osteoporosis as your susceptibility will depend on the amount of bone mass built up during chidhood and young adulthood. This can depend on genetics and diet. Black women, for instance, build up greater bone mass than do Asian or white women. The gene which is involved in the control of bone density has recently been discovered and this could lead to great advances in the prevention and treatment of osteoporosis.

SELF-HELP

At the moment, the best advice for preventing osteoporosis is as follows:
- Give up smoking.
- Keep within the recommended alcohol limits for women of 21 units a week.
  (The good news is that moderate drinking may actually be beneficial, so there's no need for total abstention.)
- Take up exercise (see Chapter 7).
- Follow a healthy diet (see Chapter 7).
- Be aware of the warning signs. If you have already broken a bone

after a minor bump or fall you may already have osteoporosis. Other warning signs include a loss in height and kyphosis, or curvature of the spine.

MEDICAL HELP

If you are worried or if you are thinking of using HRT as a preventative measure, it's worth talking to your doctor about screening. Most doctors agree that, if there are no risk factors involved and you are happy with the decision to take HRT, a bone density test is not necessary. There are no dangers to the screening process, but it is costly and it is not yet known whether it is effective in predicting whether you will suffer fractures or not. One doctor described it in terms of taking a blood pressure reading to test for hypertension. It shows a risk factor for a heart attack, but doesn't necessarily mean you will have one. Similarly, the current test can show a drop in bone density, but is not believed accurately to predict whether or not you will suffer fractures. A long-term study of screening is in progress, but has not yet reported on the effectiveness or otherwise of scanning.

If you are considered high risk your doctor may recommend you go for a scan which can establish whether you have osteoporosis or not. It can also be useful in measuring the effects of any treatment. A Dual Energy X-Ray Absorptiometry (DXA) scan using low doses of radiation is used to measure the density of the bones. You are asked to lie down on a machine for 10 to 15 minutes whilst an X-ray arm passes over you to take an image of the spine and hip. Some centres measure the density of the wrist. In some areas of the country access to scanners is limited, so if your doctor has identified a fracture on a normal X-ray or if risk factors are high you may be given treatment without a scan. If you really want one, you can pay for it privately, but the National Osteoporosis Society emphasises that, if you do choose to get your own scan done, you must have it interpreted by an expert. There are other possible tests for the future which are currently being researched. One involves a urine test which would look for biochemical markers, another involves ultrasound.

We'll discuss the latest research on HRT and its role in prevention and treatment of osteoporosis in the next two chapters. If you don't want to take HRT, you may find the following helpful.

SERMs

These are selective oestrogen receptor modulators. The most common is raloxifene, usually prescribed under the brand name Evista. It may be useful for at-risk women who cannot tolerate HRT. It is discussed more fully in Chapters 4 and 5.

Biphosphonates

These are non-hormonal drugs which work by slowing down the cells which break down bone (osteoclasts) enabling the bone-building cells (osteoblasts) to work more effectively and increase bone density. Currently there are two used to treat osteoporosis.

- Alendronate is licensed for osteoporosis treatment in post-menopausal women. It can increase bone density and reduce the risk of fractures. Benefits begin within a year and increase in the second and third years. After that there are minimal improvements, but long-term use is probably necessary for long-term protection. Alendronate can have side-effects on the digestive system, including nausea, indigestion and occasional inflammation of the oesophagus. To combat these effects it has to be taken on an empty stomach.

- Etidronate is licensed for prevention of osteoporosis in women with low bone density and treatment of the disease in post-menopausal women. It's taken in a three-month cycle with a prescribed calcium supplement. Like alendronate, it can also affect the digestive system.

New biphosphonates are currently being developed and tested.

Calcitonin

This is a hormone produced by the thyroid gland which reduces the bone dissolving activity of the osteoclasts and can be given on prescription as a treatment for osteoporosis after the menopause. It improves bone density and reduces the likelihood of fractures, although it is not as effective as HRT or biphosphonates. It is not often prescribed as it can only be given by injection, but uniquely, it can relieve the pain of recent fractures in the spine.

Calcium

This will be dealt with in full in Chapter 7.

URINARY PROBLEMS AND INCONTINENCE

Which of us hasn't coughed, laughed, jumped about in an aerobics class or run for a bus and thought, 'Whoops?' Well, maybe some of you haven't, but you are the self-righteous so-and-sos who somehow found the time in the throes of early motherhood to do those pelvic floor exercises religiously. Most of us didn't – and, boy, do we regret it now. Do pass this on to your daughters. If anyone had bothered to tell me just why I should be spending the time (i.e. it wasn't just for my partner's benefit in the short term, but mine in the long term) I might have taken it a bit more seriously.

Reliable figures on how many of us suffer and to what degree are difficult to obtain because we tend not to discuss it either with each other or our medical practitioners, but it's estimated that two out of every five women will suffer some form of weakness. For most of us it's an occasional problem and can be fixed by finally getting round to those exercises. For some of us it's so bad that it can be seriously restrictive, affecting both work and social life. And that's when you go to the doctor. No point in suffering damply in silence.

The causes of urge incontinence or stress incontinence can be a weakening of the pelvic floor muscles or a decrease in the sensitivity of the nerves at the neck of the bladder. Prolapse of the womb can also cause problems, as can infections and cystitis.

RISK FACTORS

Incontinence is more common in women who have had children – and didn't do their pelvic floor exercises properly!

SELF-HELP

- For infections, drinking lots of water is a help as is cranberry juice. Cut down on booze, tea and coffee.
- If the trouble is incontinence, you should relax, rather than straining to empty the bladder, and try not to hold back for too long or go too often as the bladder can contract.
- Do the exercises: if you don't have any infection, halfway through a wee, stop the stream, hold for a second and then let it go again. Whenever you're sitting – knitting, reading, working at the keyboard – spend a few minutes tightening and lifting it all up – vagina, bottom, pelvic floor muscles – and letting go again. No one can see from your face what you're up to and you'll be surprised how quickly the condition improves.

MEDICAL HELP

- Surgery for prolapse as outlined earlier under hysterectomy.
- Weighted vaginal cones may be recommended to improve the strength of the muscles (you just have to keep them from falling out!) and electrical stimulation techniques.
- There are new medicines available to stabilise the bladder wall.
- HRT may have a helpful effect.
- Surgery to tuck and tighten.

BREAST CANCER

Is there any one of us who doesn't have a friend or relative who has had breast cancer and doesn't fear it for herself? There's talk of an epidemic, but we have to keep it in proportion. It is true that more women develop breast cancer than any other type of malignancy and 30,000 new cases are diagnosed each year, but the figure that's always bandied about which says that 1 in 12 of us will get breast cancer is unnecessarily frightening. As a damned statistic which isn't quite a lie, it does give a misleading impression that vast numbers of us are dicing with death every second of our lives. In fact it refers to the risk a new-born baby girl has of developing breast cancer by the age of around 90. The risk increases with age – under 30, it's 1 in 200,000. By the age of 50, it's 1 in 200 and then 1 in 30 at the age of 75.

RISK FACTORS

The causes of breast cancer are really not known, although you are thought to be at a slightly higher risk if:

- your periods start early and end late. Thus there may be double the risk of developing breast cancer in those women who have menopause after the age of 55. It's believed to be because of longer exposure to the woman's own oestrogen. The hormone increases cell division and consequently the chances of abnormal cells developing. It may also accelerate the growth of abnormal cancer cells once they are established.
- you became pregnant after the age of 30 or never had children
- you have had benign breast lumps which showed cell changes called atypical hyperplasia. If this is the case you may need to have more regular checks in future
- you are overweight as a result of a diet high in saturated fat
- you are a heavy drinker. Smoking is thought to be a factor here too as with every other health problem under the sun
- you took the pill (a slight increase in risk), although after 10 years of being pill-free, the risk is the same as for someone who has never taken it
- you take HRT (a slightly raised risk). Thus after the age of 50, for the next 20 years, there is a 1 in 22 chance of developing breast cancer without HRT, it's 1 in 20 if you take HRT for ten years. (Don't confuse this with the 1 in 200 statistic mentioned earlier for a woman of 50 – what I'm discussing here is risk over 20 years, not at a specific age.) If you carry on with HRT over 15 years the risk goes up to 1 in 17 or 1 in 18. Recent studies have shown, though, that HRT seems to have an influence only in the type of slow growing and treatable cancer which is the most common type found in older women. There is no evidence that it exacerbates the fast-growing, rapidly lethal types. (More on this in Chapter 5)
- you have a family history of breast cancer, where several members of the family have had the disease (a possible genetic connection)

SELF-HELP

Whilst it's as well to be 'breast aware', which means checking your breasts regularly for any lumps or thickening, change in outline, puckering or dimpling of the skin or soreness around the nipple which looks like dermatitis or eczema – in fact anything that is new for you and is not felt in the other breast – there is no point in wasting your healthy life worrying about what might never happen. I'm always a bit wary of men who tell women, 'It is possible to have too much cancer awareness' as Professor Michael Baum, one of the leading specialists in the field did in 1997, but it is worth remembering that nine out of ten breast lumps are found to be benign and I could list for you a number of friends, some under, some over 50, who have developed breast cancer, been treated successfully and gone on to lead long, healthy and happy lives. Half of all women who develop breast cancer will live out their normal life expectancy. Even the writer Fanny Burney, whose mastectomy (removal of the breast) was carried out in the 18th century *with no anaesthetic*, lived on for another 20 years to the age of 80. Treatments, although not necessarily pleasant these days, are certainly not as ghastly as that.

If you do find an abnormality, go to the doctor and get it checked out. If you're fobbed off, push for action. There are too many doctors who have sent a patient home with a breezy, 'It's nothing to worry about' when the patient knew in her heart there was something more serious. The health service may not be geared up for it, but, in my view, every lump is worth quick, specialist investigation. It can save lives or at least set minds at rest if there really is nothing wrong.

MEDICAL HELP

There's been a huge amount of controversy in recent years about mammography – an X-ray of the breasts that can show up tiny changes in breast tissue which would not be spotted on self-examination and may not even be felt by a doctor during a routine examination.

In Britain all women between the ages of 50 and 64 are invited for breast screening every three years. There is a pilot project to determine whether this should be extended to 69 and, in October 2000, there was pressure for it to be offered to all older women from 50 onwards. One cancer specialist estimates this would prolong the life expectancy of some 2000 women over 70 each year. Given the rise in risk as we grow older, this would seem to make sense. Screening is not offered routinely to women under the age of 50, primarily because the density of breast tissue in young women makes it more difficult to detect small cancers. Another pilot programme is in progress to assess whether this age group should be included.

Out of every 10,000 women who are screened, approximately 700 will be recalled, 100 will have a biopsy to test whether any lump found does have cancerous cells and approximately 55 of those will be found to have cancer.

Professor Baum has been one of the most fierce opponents of the breast screening programme. His critique appears pretty brutal as it seems to be based on financial considerations. On a current cost benefit analysis, he concludes that women would do better if the money invested on screening were put into hiring more breast cancer specialists. The majority of lumps he sees, he says, are detected by chance in the bath or by a partner, not by mammogram. He also says that women who get specialist treatment do best. He believes, as I have already suggested, that the best breast cancer awareness campaign would tell women to demand that their GPs refer them to breast cancer specialists and not a 'general surgeon who happens to be the GP's golfing buddy'.

New evidence came out in September 2000 which suggests the

screening programme is more useful than Professor Baum might wish to acknowledge in detecting those small cancers which are operable and can be treated with radiation or with drugs such as chemotherapy or Tamoxifen. There was a 21 per cent fall in deaths from breast cancer among women aged 55 to 69 between 1990 and 1998. Seven per cent of that fall is attributed to screening and amounts to 1000 women a year.

Whilst Baum is correct when he says that some women with the most fast-growing and invasive cancers will die no matter how early they are detected or whatever treatment they receive – he cites Linda McCartney as an example of this type of tumour – there are other types of cancer which can benefit from early detection and treatment. It is certainly easier to conserve the breast if the lump is small when treated – not an insignificant concern for any of us, no matter how old we are. In an ideal world surgeons and screening programmes would not have to compete for money – clearly we need both – although at present there are not nearly enough oncologists in this or any other field of cancer care.

The best policy, it seems to me, is to press for investigation if you think it's necessary. Julietta Patnick, who heads the National Screening Programme, told Radio 4's *Today* programme in October 2000 that no woman would be turned away if she requested a mammogram, regardless of her age. If you have a positive result you should then discuss, with a breast cancer specialist, the best kind of treatment for you. If you fall apart because you're feeling frightened, get a husband, partner, relative or friend to pitch in with you to get the best out of the NHS.

There's also been fierce debate among women about whether we want these regular tests – the pap smear for cervical cancer has come under similar scrutiny – which keep us in the clutches of the medical profession, constantly anxious about whether next time we'll be told there's something horribly wrong with us. Some commentators have compared it with the way pregnancy and childbirth have been hi-jacked by the medical profession to the extent that none of us can feel that having a baby or going through menopause might be a perfectly natural event.

In *The Menopause Industry*, Sandra Coney, describes in detail how she was 'caught up in the system' and the dilemma with which we're all faced. Here's an edited version:

> After I had been taking the HRT off and on for a year, my GP suggested it would be a good thing to get a 'baseline mammography' against which any subsequent changes in my breasts could be measured. In the end I went ahead, as much out of curiosity about the procedure as anything. The radiographer said the radiologist would look at the X-rays and send a report to the GP and I went away and promptly forgot about it.
>
> It turned out that the report did note an area of density in one of my breasts which the radiologist thought might require further examination. I asked my GP to read me the report which stated reassuringly that there were no indications of malignancy. The comment on the unexplained dense patch seemed to me to be implying that there was only the most outside chance that it might be hiding a tumour.
>
> I told her that I had no faith in mammography as a diagnostic tool and that on the basis of the report I was prepared to do nothing. She was not prepared to let the matter rest. We agreed that she should send the X-rays to a breast specialist.
>
> The specialist did want to see me and he wanted me to have some more mammograms done. He also wanted me to have an ultrasound scan. It occurred to me to tell him that it was not me who was worrying, but my GP, but I thought better of it.
>
> I went out to the specialist clutching a big envelope of X-rays. After examining the new X-rays and the ultrasound report, and giving my breasts a thorough examination, the specialist told me

there did not seem to be anything there he could do a biopsy on. He did not think it was anything to be concerned about, but just to be on the safe side, I should go for another mammogram in six months. That would be one year after the first one. I was convinced that the whole effort was a case of over-treatment. But I got hooked into a system which threatened me, both implicitly and explicitly, with the risk of death if I did not comply. I am tempted to let it slip. I know I am at low risk for breast cancer. In terms of all the risk factors in my life and history I am more likely to die of heart disease. But there is always an outside chance that they are right and I am wrong.

Coney believed she was coerced into paying privately for her investigations, having been advised by the specialist that it would take a long time to get an appointment in one of New Zealand's public hospitals and there may be a question here of whether too many investigations are done in the private system because of the profit motive. Nevertheless, it is easy to see how we can end up in a spiral of worry which may do us harm. Equally, there is concern about the number of X-rays delivered if repeated tests are carried out. Some people will argue that even the small dose delivered by a mammogram carries its own risk.

In the end, it's up to us to choose. I went through a similar process to Coney's in the summer of 2000. Having volunteered to take part in a study of natural progesterone, I had, as part of the trial, to have a full MOT to establish my state of health before the trial, so that any changes could be monitored and reported. After the mammogram I had a phone call on my mobile. I was in Tesco's, not the best place to be told there was 'an irregularity on the mammogram'. I went a bit wobbly and pale, arranged to go for further investigations within the week and then put it to the back of my mind.

At the hospital I was given an ultrasound scan, rather like the one you have when you're pregnant, was told there were definitely lumps, probably not malignant, but it might be a good idea to have a needle biopsy. The radiologist could do it right away if I wanted. I did. I was warned it was marginally worse than the dentist, but couldn't be done with an anaesthetic as the area to be numbed is too large. (Compliments, compliments. One unexpected result of my menopause has been a significant increase in chest measurement. It makes a change from the days when I was the most flat-chested girl in the school, known as Peanut!)

Whether my practitioner was particularly good at her job or not, I don't know, but it was nothing. I hardly felt the needle go in. There was a bit of a funny feeling as it wiggled about, although it wasn't painful. The radiologist watches what she's doing on the screen, sucks out stuff from the lump, repeats the whole process from another position and you're away. Results were promised in two or three days. I felt a bit shaky, so I treated myself to a very expensive lunch in a restaurant just around the corner (including a bottle of wine). It was after I sobered up that I began to panic and I was terrified by the time the results came through. Negative. Just cysts, nothing at all to worry about. So I've been through the trauma of being a statistical false positive and for a short time I was indeed converted from a well woman into a worried one. Frankly, for me, it was worth it, possibly irrationally, to know that, for now at least, I'm all clear. But then, hypochondria is my middle name.

Janet Balaskas, founder of the Active Birth Movement, had a similar experience to mine. She chose to pay a private gynae-cologist to check her breasts and did not have a mammogram, only a highly sophisticated ultrasound scan. Her gynaecologist chose not to use mammography because of slight concerns that the X-rays used may be carcinogenic and also felt the ultrasound would give a more detailed picture. Janet's story of how she got rid of her cysts is told in Chapter 6.

CERVICAL CANCER

Many of these same arguments have been tossed around over the cervical screening programme, which was set up under the instigation of Edwina Currie, when she was health minister and has been running since the late 1980s. Under the current system all women between the ages of 20 and 64 are invited for a smear test every three or five years. There have been a number of scandals about both false positives and negatives, usually because of errors by a single individual in taking the samples, reading the results or because of poor performance in the laboratory.

Cervical cancer is relatively rare. The most recent figures show there were 2740 new cases in England and Wales in 1997, which is a 26 per cent fall in incidence over the previous five years. The Imperial Cancer Research Fund claims that cervical screening prevents between 1000 and 3900 cases each year.

Ruth Lea of the Institute of Directors threw a huge spanner in the works in the spring of 2000, when she produced a contradictory report saying that the government's own statisitics showed screening cost £120 million a year and saved only 800 lives. Her suggestion was that mass screening should be scrapped and scarce NHS funds spent on greater priorities.

One of her main objections to the scheme, as she told *The Times*, is that 'the wrong women are screened. Cervical cancer is related to – not to put too fine a point on it – sexual promiscuity.' And of course, to some degree, she's right. The primary cause of cervical cancer is the human papilloma virus (HPV), a sexually transmitted disease. Promiscuity, though, is a bit of an exaggeration. Some of us might have picked up the virus in our twenties when the pill was all the rage and we hadn't yet got to the point where we'd passed sexual liberation, which gave us the right to say yes, and moved on to women's liberation which made it OK to say no. And, let's face it, some of us had a high old time, entirely without shame or guilt. Other women, though, may have led monogamous lives, but their husbands haven't, or they may have performed one small indiscretion themselves and caught the virus.

I can see why it was important in the 1980s to tread carefully on women's sensibilities to encourage them to come forward for the test. I like to think that now we are not so coy as to have to pretend that the majority of us, male and female, have had only one sexual partner throughout our lives and we can be honest about telling women what the real risks are. If you're a non-smoking virgin, you may decide you are not too worried and choose not to attend when called for screening. If you're not, it seems to me to make sense to have the test. Stay calm if you're recalled – a positive result does not necessarily mean you have cancer. It could be the smear wasn't carried out correctly, or the lab may have messed up, or it may be that the abnormalities shown may be pre-cancerous. If further tests do show pre-cancerous or cancerous cells, treatment is usually successful. A new screening programme which will specifically look for HPV is now being piloted. Treatment for the virus, it's hoped, will prevent the majority of cases of cervical cancer from developing.

Ruth Lea admits she has a personal objection to the progamme. She believes her risk of contracting the virus and, consequently, the cancer, is very low, and is furious that she was not told the truth about her level of risk and given the opportunity to choose whether to have the test or not. If we didn't have to, none of us would choose to lie with our legs apart whilst a GP does unspeakable things with a chilly speculum and spatula and Ruth is resentful that she dutifully went along when called, when she believes that in her case it was probably unnecessary. She's concerned, too, that paying doctors for each test performed damages the doctor–patient relationship. She rightly asks, 'What incentive is there for a doctor to discuss the pros and cons for each individual when he or she is effectively paid for every slide sent off to the lab?' The experience has shaken her confidence in the medical profession. (There's more of Ruth's story in Chapter 6 on complementary treatments.)

So, I guess the upshot of this chapter is that it's not a particularly wise move to put your trust in your doctor blindly. Be well informed, ask lots of questions and press for the treatment you want. (See p. 283 for details of helpful and authoritative organisations.) Your good health should come as a result of a partnership between you and your medical practitioner. Gone are the days when the old joke was passed around the waiting room. What's the difference between God and a doctor? God doesn't think he (or she) is a doctor!

CHAPTER 4

WHAT IS HRT?

People often ask me who, from the hundreds, nay thousands, of people I've interviewed over the years, was the most impressive. Easy. Bette Davis. It was early in my career on *Woman's Hour*, she had written an autobiography and was holding court at the Savoy, deigning to allow certain selected journalists half an hour of her time. Waiting with me in the lobby was the *grande dame* of Fleet Street, Jean Rook, and even she was terrified at the prospect of being mauled by a screen legend.

Davis was frightening, known for her tendency to tear limb from limb any journalist to whom she took a dislike. She was nearly 80, tiny and a little stiff in her movements, but impeccably dressed in a neat black number, immaculately made up, coiffed and manicured. Her eyes bored through you, searching for insincerity and, when she found genuine interest and (preferably) adoration, she gave a wonderful interview, explaining how as a young woman she had learned always to look like a movie star – it was what her fans expected, and being old made no difference to her professionalism. At the end of our conversation I told her my favourite moment in the movies is in *All About Eve*, where, standing on the stairs as the ageing actress Margo Channing, she delivers the line 'Fasten your seatbelts, it's gonna be a bumpy night!' Davis did the line for me, following it with that sly smile of

hers and her smoky, throaty laugh. Some months later she died, a
great star to the last.

It's strange that she and that famous line should come to mind
as I embarked on these chapters about HRT. 'Fasten your seatbelts,
it's gonna be a bumpy night!' I don't know whether she took it, I
would never have dared to ask, but I was as scared of starting on
this work as I was of her. My fears about giving advice on the
therapy were echoed in June 2000 by an American journalist,
Kathleen MacAuliffe, who was writing for the *New York Times*
about the research into the new ultra low-dose hormone therapies.
'Nowadays,' she said, 'it seems as if only people with a PhD in
epidemiology – and preferably circus experience – can juggle all
the pros and cons of HRT, much less make sense of all the
conflicting reports.'

I confess to having neither qualification and am in much the
same position as you. I'm an ordinary woman, with some
journalistic and communication skills, trying to make up my own
mind about what will make the third part of my life as healthy,
useful and enjoyable as were the first two. The research I've done
is as much for my benefit as yours. In the end, it's simply about
sifting through what appears to be a medical minefield, of
inconclusive research and fierce disagreements, and then making
up our own minds on the basis of what risks and benefits we're
prepared to balance in our own lives!

It's estimated that around 25 per cent of women over the age of
45 are taking HRT and, amongst women doctors, the figure is
thought to be more than 40 per cent. The Million Women Study
results show that of women aged 50 to 64 in the UK half have used
hormone replacement therapy at some time and a third of women
in the age group are currently taking the treatment.

Dr Marion Everitt, who runs the Menopause Clinic in Leeds, is
a fan. She says she became irritable in her mid-forties and began to
have hot sweats which were a professional embarrassment. She,

you may remember, has no difficulty in seeing menopause as a deficiency disease to be treated with hormones in much the same way as you would treat diabetes with insulin, but her experience with clients and with her own treatment has demonstrated the need to tailor carefully the right dose and method of delivery for the individual woman. In her own case she tried patches which kept falling off, took three types of tablet which gave her headaches, then finally hit on a gel that delivers the oestrogen she needs and a Mirena (progestogen coil) that gives her the progestogen she requires.

Women like Teresa Gorman, Jo Wagerman and Joan Bakewell have been taking HRT for many years, from their forties, when they first had symptoms of the menopause, into their sixties, adjusting type and dose as new products have come on the market or their needs have changed. Each of them is convinced that HRT helps to maintain their feeling of well-being. Some women take it for a short while to deal with the worst symptoms of the menopause and then give up because they don't want to take medication for the rest of their lives. The medical journalist, Lesley Hilton, after a number of unpleasant run-ins with patches, discovered through trial and error a mixture of oestrogen and low progestogen in tablet form which she uses when she really feels she needs to. One summer, for instance, she booked a holiday in Greece and couldn't face hot flushes in the heat, so she decided to take the HRT, just to keep her comfy on holiday.

Some women find that HRT doesn't suit them at all. They give it a go, decide they hate it and give it up almost at once. Eve Pollard, the former newspaper and magazine editor, now novelist, is one. Eve tells me she never got on with oestrogen. She tried the pill as a contraceptive years ago and says she felt she was going to explode almost before she left the doctor's surgery. She jokes about the ample chest for which she's always been well known and explains she really didn't need to feel it was being augmented.

When, during her perimenopause in her early fifties, she began to have mild symptoms of sleeplessness and then her periods stopped, she thought perhaps she should do something and tried an HRT implant. She found the oestrogen in the HRT had the same bloating effect as the pill. It made her feel, she says, as if 'it wasn't me'. As she's now relatively symptom-free, she's wondering about other methods of helping her bones and skin to stay healthy, without having to bother with HRT (see Chapter 6).

As HRT is such a big and complex subject, I've split it into two chapters. This one simply endeavours to explain what HRT is, where it comes from and what it claims to achieve. In the next chapter we'll juggle those pros and cons and try to keep all the balls in the air!

HRT, or Hormone Replacement Therapy, refers to drugs which provide forms of oestrogen alone or combined drugs that deliver forms of oestrogen and progesterone. Oestrogen alone is given to women who have had a hysterectomy and consequently have no uterus but, to reduce the risk of endometrial cancer in women who do have a womb, progestogens are given to 'oppose' the effect of oestrogen, as they do in a normal menstrual cycle, preventing the lining of the womb from being overstimulated.

If you have a womb, modern HRT mimics the menstrual cycle. Oestrogen is given every day of the month and a progestogen is added for 10 to 14 days each month. About 85 per cent of women will have a monthly bleed, although there are now 'no-bleed' HRTs for women who are post-menopausal.

In general, HRT replaces oestrogen to about two-thirds of premenopausal levels, with the intention of slowing down the changes accelerated by the menopause, rather than arresting the ageing process altogether. Short-term use, as we've discussed, can provide symptomatic relief of hot flushes and night sweats. Moyra Livesey from the Rylstone WI calendar had dreadful night sweats and put up with them for four or five months, thinking it was only neurotic and needy women who would suffer symptoms. Believing herself to be sensible, well-adjusted and well-informed, she buried her head in the sand until the problems became too hard to bear. The night sweats got worse and she became quite depressed and miserable, with no energy. She worried that her brain was going to mush and made lists all the time to remind her what she was supposed to be doing. Worst of all, she was horrible to her teenage son. It was so consistently bad, she says, she couldn't explain it away as 'just having a bad day'.

Moyra's GP was reluctant to prescribe HRT as there was some breast cancer in the family, so instead she talked to her daughter, who is also a GP. She convinced her mum that the family breast cancer was not genetic and told her to have a blood test. When her hormone levels were found to be low, Moyra went away and weighed up the pros and cons, took alternatives for a while and then, like Lesley Hilton, opted for HRT in desperation before a holiday. She and her husband had booked to go sailing in Turkey and she knew hot flushes and night sweats would be unbearable in the confined space of a boat. In what she describes as a 'total panic' she went to the doctor and began a course of combined HRT in tablet form. The improvements happened, she says 'amazingly quickly – within four or five days – I can hardly believe how quickly I felt better'. She's 51, doing well and has no plans to come off the tablets. She's convinced that taking the therapy long-term will help her to combat heart disease and osteoporosis (more details in Chapter 5).

WHAT'S IN HRT

The point of HRT is that it replaces the oestrogen that is lost as women go through the menopause and beyond. It's not, of course, as easy as simply putting the same substance that we produce ourselves into a tablet form, because hormones have to get past the enzymes and acids in the stomach and into the bloodstream whilst remaining biologically active. They then have to get through the liver (known as the 'first pass') before entering the main circulation system to get on with their work.

The blood in the body is constantly circulating through the liver so that unwanted substances can be cleared. The kidneys do a similar filtering job, so we need repeated doses of the drugs to keep levels up. The molecular structure of the hormones has to be robust enough to get through all the filters (our own oestrogen, taken orally, would be fought off as an invader!) and doses have to be high enough so that, even if some of the drug is destroyed, it still has an effect. When the active ingredient does get through, it still has to fit the hormone receptors to have the desired result. Thus, replacement therapy, whilst not the same as that produced by the body, must have a related structure if it's to work effectively.

OESTROGENS

The female body naturally produces three types of oestrogen:
- oestradiol
- oestrone
- oestriol

Oestradiol is the primary oestrogen produced by the ovaries. Oestrone is formed from oestradiol. It is a weak oestrogen and is the most abundant oestrogen found in the body after menopause. Oestriol is produced in large quantities during pregnancy and is a breakdown product of oestradiol.

Oestradiol – the strongest of the three – doesn't get through the gut lining very well, but it can be manufactured in a micronised form, which means it is broken down into tiny particles, which the gut finds easier to absorb. Some tablets contain substances which are related, but are more easily absorbed. So the ingredients on a pack of HRT might include oestradiol valerate or piperazine oestrone sulphate. Other tablets use oestriol or a combination of all three. Some of these oral oestrogens are converted to oestrone by the time they reach the bloodstream – and it's worth noting that this means that blood oestradiol levels taken by doctors after a course of HRT has begun may not be a true representation of the level of hormones in the body at any one time. A complete break of at least three months is necessary to check the body's own baseline.

Edwina Currie pointed to this as a difficulty in trying to find the right HRT for her. For the first three months she took quite a high dose of both oestrogen and progestogen. The high dose of progestogen made her feel edgy and more feisty than usual (a side-effect she really didn't need!). She also felt her libido was raised to unacceptable levels (some of us might not complain about that!) and she began to look like a spotty teenager as it gave her a kind of acne. She had blood tests to pick up the levels of oestrogen in her system which have consistently been found to be similar to those in pre-menopausal women. The test, she thinks, is not as refined as it could be and it is, of course, difficult, during replacement therapy, to distinguish what is the body's own level of oestradiol or oestrone and what has been converted from the HRT. Edwina preferred to find the right dose by trial and error. Now she's settled for Premarin tablets with a standard oestrogen dose of 0.625mg, and takes a lower dose of progestogen. She's happy taking tablets as she got used to it over years of taking the pill and she feels well, her skin is good and her temperament much calmer.

There are salivary hormone tests which are more reliable than the blood test. Even though this is a better way of measuring, it is still, in the opinion of some doctors, misleading as there is no optimum oestrogen level for any woman, only the level which makes you feel well. Again, trial and error to establish the right dose for you and to deal with your symptoms seems to be the only way of getting it right. Most specialists monitor on symptom control with visual analogue scores of symptom ratings and quality of the questionnaires.

'Natural' oestrogens

The different oestrogen preparations used in HRT are known as 'natural oestrogens' because, even though they are artificially manufactured in the laboratory, from plant substances found in soya beans or cacti or from the urine of pregnant mares, they contain or give rise to the same oestrogens naturally produced in the female body.

In *The Menopause, HRT and You*, Caroline Hawkridge, points out that the word 'natural' has been used as an advertiser's dream, second only to the word 'new'. We shouldn't be fooled into believing that the word 'natural' when used to describe hormones in HRT is the equivalent of what we would naturally produce in the wild. As we've seen, it's horse urine – a natural product – which gives the closest animal oestrogen to that found in humans. Oestrogens derived from plants could also be said to be 'natural', but can only be made to work in the human female after they've been synthesised in the laboratory. Drugs are drugs, and no medical therapy can really be described as natural, whatever its source. But then it isn't 'natural' to dye the hair, swathe the skin in anti-wrinkle cream or take aspirin for a headache, yet most of us do it anyway. I just prefer not to have the wool pulled over my eyes by clever marketing. (*Note*: There are other types of natural oestrogen known as phyto-oestrogens, which will be covered in Chapter 6.)

Equine oestrogen

Premarin is the brand name of one of the most popular forms of HRT, but it has caused a great deal of unease amongst animal rights campaigners because, as its name suggests, it is derived from the urine of pregnant mares. Prempak and Premique are also produced in this way. Conjugated equine oestrogens are a mixture of 50 to 65 per cent oestrone sulphate and the horse oestrogen, equilin sulphate. It has a similar structure to human oestrogens and works well with the oestrogen receptors.

Some doctors are more keen on equine oestrogen than others. A menopause GP, Annie Evans, says its rich mixture is complex and the effects of the ingredients vary, and Andrew Prentice, a gynaecologist I spoke to, told me he preferred to prescribe more modern HRTs. Nevertheless, Val Godfree of the Amarant Trust menopause advisory service points out it remains one of the market leaders despite the emergence of new products during the 50 years it has been around and several million women worldwide can't be wrong!

You may, of course, have concerns about the animals. Horse Aid, a pressure group, says on its website that there are 600 farms in Canada producing Pregnant Mare's Urine (PMU) and about 40 in the USA. They claim that horses are kept tied up indoors for at least six months of the year. They say they are impregnated and fitted with a painful catheter-type 'urine collection device', then normally kept indoors for the 11 months of their pregnancy, in stalls 8ft by 3ft 6 in by 5ft. In some cases, according to Horse Aid, they are artificially inseminated within two weeks of foaling and are returned to the 'production line'. The foal is removed and said to be sold for slaughter. Horse Aid agree that catheters are no longer used to collect the urine, but claim that the new devices are unhygienic and allow the urine to soak into the skin of the mares.

The North American Equine Ranching Information Council (NAERIC) says the mares are turned out to pasture in March ready for foaling in May. In June, stallions are introduced to the pastures to run with mares and foals and breeding takes place over the next two months. Stallions are removed in August and mares and foals remain at grass until the foals are weaned, some time after 1

September. The urine collection season runs from mid-October to mid-March, when the cycle begins again. NAERIC say the urine collection devices allow for free movement of the horse within the stall and are not irritating. Wyeth Ayerst, the company which produces the drugs from the urine, says the mares would be kept indoors throughout winter anyway because of the severe weather conditions in Canada and North America. The company says it has its own team of inspectors which checks on the stock on the farms and demands that farmers stick to a Code of Practice. The company also says foals are sold for riding, showing, breeding or other sports. No mention is made of the meat trade.

I haven't checked out the farms for myself and would not presume to sway you either way. Those are the 'facts' from both sides. It's up to you and there are other types of therapy to choose from if you have objections to the kind of 'natural' HRT that requires horses to be farmed in this way.

Synthetic oestrogens

These include substances such as ethinyloestradiol, mestranol and stilboestrol, all used in the contraceptive pill. They are called 'synthetic' because the body can't convert them into the same substances it produces naturally. The doses are more concentrated than those used in HRT and need to be potent enough to prevent the ovaries from producing an egg each month. This is the contraceptive effect which prevents pregnancy in a fertile woman. In fact, the pill uses oestrogens which are up to eight times more potent than 'natural' oestrogens. Almost all HRT contains 'natural oestrogens'.

Synthetics in the form of the contraceptive pill are sometimes prescribed for younger women who have problem periods, but long-term use can bring a bigger risk of high blood pressure and blood clots than is generally associated with HRT. Synthetic oestrogens can make the blood more sticky.

Thus the main differences between the contraceptive pill and HRT are:

The contraceptive pill
- contains 'synthetic' oestrogens
- contains high doses of oestrogens
- increases the risk of blood clot and thrombosis

HRT
- usually contains 'natural' oestrogens
- has low doses of oestrogen
- has a lower risk of blood clots and thrombosis

Consequently, some women who are unable to take the contraceptive pill because of certain risk factors or because they feel unwell on high doses of synthetic oestrogen may be able to consider taking HRT.

PROGESTERONE

The body produces only one form of its own progesterone, but if this is ingested or absorbed by any other method than the body's own means of production it is easily dismantled by the body before it has a chance to work on the progesterone receptors. So HRT tends to contain related compounds called *progestogens*. These are biochemically modified versions of progesterone which are less easily destroyed and can work on the body's receptors.

Oral natural progesterone is available and is used more in France than in the UK, but because such high doses need to be taken, it needs to be administered twice a day. As we saw from Edwina Currie's experience, high doses of progestogens can cause unpleasant side-effects. Acne, water retention, weight gain, breast discomfort and pre-menstrual symptoms have all been reported. One of the biggest problems with natural proesterone is that it induces drowsiness. Progesterone suppositories and a vaginal gel called Crinone (see below) are also available.

'Natural progesterone' cream, derived from wild yam and synthesised in the laboratory has been much touted as an alternative to HRT. I'll discuss it fully in Chapter 6.

The common progestogens found in most HRT preparations are of two types:

Progestogens derived from progesterone (known as C21 progestogens):
- dydrogesterone
- medroxyprogesterone acetate

Progestogens derived from testosterone (known as C19 progestogens):
- levnorgestrel
- norethisterone
- norgestrel

Methods of Taking HRT

HRT can be given in various forms, including pills, patches, implants, gels and sprays. You will need to weigh up the pros and cons of each, to decide which method is best for you.

Pills

These, as we've seen, can be oestrogen alone (for women who have had a hysterectomy) or combined oestrogen and progestogen.

Oestrogen is taken on a daily basis with no break. Different tablets contain different forms and amounts. Some are a fixed dose, whereas others mimic the ups and downs of the menstrual cycle, but this has no real advantage in symptomatic relief. Pills can be given in two forms: sequential combined HRT, and continuous combined or 'no-bleed' HRT.

Sequential combined HRT

Oestrogen and progestogen is taken as 'sequential combined HRT', where oestrogen tablets are taken every day and progestogen for 10–14 days a month. These may be in a calendar pack, like the pill, or, if there isn't a combined form which suits you, the oestrogen may come in the pack and you may be given progestogen from a different preparation or by a different method of delivery.

When the progestogen is finished and levels fall, the lining of the womb is shed as a 'period' or more accurately a 'withdrawal bleed'. The amount of blood lost varies. It may be only a little and about 15 per cent of women have no blood loss at all. The television and radio presenter Joan Bakewell, now in her mid-sixties, is one of that small percentage who don't bleed on this form of HRT. She recognised her menopausal symptoms when she was 45 and put up with horrible flushes and sweats for about six months. When it really began to get her down – the flushes were beginning to spoil social events – she went to the doctor and was prescribed HRT. Reminding me that this was 20 years ago, she says the doses then were generally much higher than they are now, but she had no side-effects. Her doctor was a little worried that she had no bleeding, but monitored her carefully and found no problems. She thought it was 'great' not to have periods.

Her dosage has, she says, become 'more finely tuned' as the years have gone on and the therapy has become more sophisticated. She did once come off it, having read a 'breast cancer scare story' in the papers. Her sister, who was younger than Joan, had died of the disease and Joan was worried enough about her own health to stop. She describes the six weeks during which she didn't take HRT as 'unbelievably awful. I felt as though I was falling over all the time.' She weighed up the balance of risks versus benefits, decided her

HRT was helping to keep her fit and active and now she pops her Prempak every day, keeps a close check on her breasts and has no plans to give up.

(Note: There is another form of sequential HRT called Tridestra which is designed to produce a bleed only once every three months. This is suitable for women who are less than a year past the menopause but it can have a high incidence of breakthrough bleeding while the body settles to it.)

Continuous combined HRT

Continuous combined, or 'no-bleed' HRT is a newer development that is suitable for women who are more than one year past the menopause – irregular bleeding can occur if it's used while periods are still occurring naturally. These preparations contain a daily dose of oestrogen and progestogen and this has the effect of stopping the usual monthly bleed associated with the standard HRT. It is quite common for women to have spotting or slight bleeding during the first course which may put some people off. The research indicates that women prefer not to bleed while taking HRT – which seems totally obvious to me, as being period-free is one of the great benefits of being post-menopausal. Continuous combined HRT, if you can stick with the initial hiccups, is probably the best bet if you were glad to kiss goodbye to the tampons.

Some forms of continuous combined HRT have been shown to provide superior protection against osteoporosis when compared with sequential combined HRT, probably due to the continuous dose of progestogen.

Continuous combined HRT may be helpful in reducing the symptoms of pre-menstrual syndrome, which can occur when the progestogen is added for only the second part of the month. The daily progestogen dose in continuous combined HRT is usually lower than that used with sequential therapies. There are said to be fewer side-effects such as painful breasts, fluid retention, abdominal swelling, anxiety and mood swings with this form of treatment.

Do be firm and discuss the option of 'no-bleed HRT' with your doctor. One friend of Jo Wagerman's went to hers in desperation. Her night sweats were so bad she was spending half the night on her doorstep in her nightie. When she asked her doctor about HRT she was dismissed with a, 'You don't want to be having periods when you're 90!' No, she doesn't, but then she doesn't have to. Even if you have been on sequential HRT in the perimenopausal period and are not sure whether or not your periods have stopped because of withdrawal bleeds, you can take a break once you think you might be past the menopause and then change your HRT. (This is what I plan to do after the natural progesterone trial is finished – unless it works miracles.)

Advantages

- They are easy to take and remember as, like the pill, they come in calendar packs.
- They are easily reversible.
- There are many different types to suit different women.

Disadvantages

- They need to be taken every day.
- This isn't the most natural way to deliver hormones. The oral route means doses need to be high enough to get past the liver, so a load is placed on the organ, which normally would not be asked to process such large amounts of oestrogen. Also, the level in the bloodstream varies daily, increasing after a pill is taken and then falling until the next one is taken. The high dose needed to counteract this problem can cause more side-effects such as nausea.
- There is a big variation in the amount of oestrogen absorbed from pills in different individuals. Two women taking the same

dose may have different levels in their system over and above the differences created by their own production of oestrogen.
- Some women don't like taking pills as it 'feels like medication'.
- The majority of pills contain lactose as a bulking agent and are not suitable for women with a lactose sensitivity.

PATCHES

Patches can deliver oestrogen alone for women who have had a hysterectomy. The oestrogen-only patch can be used by women who have not had a hysterectomy, but has to be opposed by progestogen pills for the necessary 10 to 14 days. Patches are also available as sequential combined HRT. This involves wearing two weeks' worth of oestrogen-only patches and two weeks of oestrogen combined with progestogen. There is a patch which delivers continuous combined HRT, but there is no progestogen-only patch. The larger the dose, the larger the patch.

The newer type of patch is called a 'matrix'. The older kind is described as a 'reservoir'. The new patches are thinner than the old-style versions and, instead of the hormone being in a reservoir in the middle, it's mixed in with the adhesive which sticks the patch to the skin. It is possible to have an adverse reaction to the alcohol contained in the reservoir-type patch or to the adhesive, although there are fewer reported problems with the matrix patch. Nevertheless, regardless of the type of patch, it is recommended that the site of the application is varied each time the patch is changed.

Some patches are changed every week, some twice a week. The oestradiol is absorbed in a steady trickle from the underside of the patch through the skin and the layer of subcutaneous fat beneath it. It goes directly into the bloodstream, avoiding the 'first pass' through the liver. It's recommended that the patch should be stuck on an area of clean, dry, unbroken skin below the waist, usually the upper part of the buttock or the thigh. It needs to be firmly held in place by the finger for ten seconds and then sealed by running the fingers around the edge.

If it comes off it can be restuck. It should stay on whilst having a bath or shower or whilst swimming, but it can be removed and then replaced. It is not advisable to wear it while sunbathing or on a sunbed as the skin can be become moist through sweating and then the patch won't stick very well.

Advantages

- The patch is a more natural means of delivery of hormones physiologically than taking pills. Doses are in micrograms rather than milligrams and, as the 'first pass' through the liver is avoided, there are likely to be fewer side effects. The hormones do eventually go through the liver and the eventual levels of hormones in the blood will be the same as with tablets, but gradual absorption means that more constant levels are maintained throughout the day.
- The resulting circulating oestrogen remains mostly as oestradiol, rather than the majority being converted to oestrone, so the levels are much closer to what might be expected in the body pre-menopause.

Disadvantages

- Skin reactions, including mild itching or redness are possible. It's worth trying different types of patches if this is the case.
- There is only one type of progestogen (Norethisterone) available at the moment in patch form and this may not be suitable for everyone.
- The patch can look unsightly and can come unstuck and start to peel off before it's time to change. One friend woke up in the middle of the night, felt for her patch and found it was missing. She scrabbled around in the bedclothes to no avail and only

discovered it the next morning stuck to her husband. Then she lost it on the floor at a party. A talking point, I suppose, but not one that everyone would welcome as a topic of conversation!

The newer patches are said to be better. Progynova TS is a weekly oestrogen patch, available in two sizes. Because it is small and transparent, it isn't very noticeable, adheres well and has a low risk of skin irritation. Nuvelle TS is a small two-phase patch which delivers both oestrogen and progestogen. It is said to provide good endometrial protection and good cycle control for women who have not had a hysterectomy.

Jo Wagerman hit on this form of HRT (she combined patch and pills) some 15 years ago and found it suited her very well. She came off the treatment just over a year ago because she had to have a hysterectomy when pre-cancerous cells were found after a smear test. During the time she was not taking HRT she says she had no drive and all her old symptoms – flushes and stiffness – came back. Her dose was changed to oestrogen only after the hysterectomy and she feels her old self again. She firmly believes that her HRT treatment has kept her free from the osteoporosis which caused her mother and grandmother to walk with sticks by the time they were 60. She also believes it helps to control the pain of her arthritis, as it was much worse when she was not using the treatment.

Lesley Hilton first took HRT when she became perimenopausal, and she too opted for patches, primarily because she was concerned that pills would deliver too high a dose and might put too much strain on the liver. Her instinct when she read the accompanying leaflet with its long list of possible side effects was to ask herself why she didn't just take a bottle of poison and have done with it. When she stuck the patch on she was sorely tempted to rip it off straight away, but her hot flushes stopped within days. She did have pre-menstrual symptoms – in fact she says she felt suicidal just before her period and found herself sobbing when she was out walking the dog. She also had agonising breast pain. She cut her patches into smaller pieces and found the side-effects diminished, but she still wasn't too happy. She allowed her dose to tail off gradually and finally gave up. The hot flushes returned.

When she decided to try HRT again to give herself a 'hot-flush holiday' she went to a local NHS specialist menopause clinic and explained the problems she had had first time around. This time she was prescribed a much lower dose of progestogen, as the doctor thought the breast pain she had experienced was probably due to too high a dose. This worked much better, although Lesley says this time the progestogen was so low that the flushes occasionally broke through, but not to a debilitating degree.

IMPLANTS

Crystalline pellets of oestradiol are inserted into the fatty tissue under the skin, usually in the lower abdomen or buttocks, and will slowly dissolve and release the oestradiol into the bloodstream. Implants generally produce the highest amounts of oestrogen of all the methods of delivery, but still within premenopausal limits.

The procedure, in which a local anaesthetic is given and the implant is injected into a small incision, can be done in a GP's surgery or a menopause clinic. Implants can also be inserted at the time of a hysterectomy. Progestogens need to be taken separately if the womb is still present.

Advantages
- They can be forgotten about for the duration of their efficacy.
- As with patches, the method is more physiologically natural than taking tablets.

Disadvantages
- A minor surgical procedure is involved.
- The implants are difficult to remove if the method doesn't suit.
- There is a risk of tachyphylaxis, or the recurrence of menopausal symptoms, while the implant is still releasing oestradiol. New implants can add to the lingering effects of old implants which gradually run out as they dissolve, but each new implant creates a sudden step up in hormone levels. The higher the levels, the sooner they drop and it's thought this sudden drop in levels, rather than the overall level of oestrogen, is what brings on the menopausal symptoms. So women can feel their implants are running out, even when their actual levels are still high. The lingering effect of the previous implants needs to be taken into account when a new one is inserted. Blood levels need to be checked before the implants are replaced and lower-dose implants used where necessary.
- When implants are no longer to be replaced, women who are taking progestogen need to continue for two or more years to counter the lingering effect of the implant.

Implants are the chosen method of delivery of HRT for Teresa Gorman, one of the most vociferous advocates of the therapy in the past few years and founder of the advisory service, the Amarant Trust. She warns of the danger of overdosing on oestrogen as an implant runs down and says she never allows herself to be tempted to have a new one inserted before the allocated time is up – in her case, every six months. She does, though, carry Oestrogel with her, which she calls 'belly jelly' (see below). She uses a little to 'top herself up' when she feels she needs it towards the end of an implant. She takes her progestogen separately and always carries both with her when she travels.

GELS

In France, oestrogen gel is the most popular form of HRT (American friends told Teresa about it, and in the early days she had to get her supplies from France. It's now available in the UK as Oestrogel and Sandrina.) It contains oestradiol in a clear gel which comes either in a canister which dispenses a measured blob or in sachets. Again, it needs to be opposed by progestogen.

Women in a natural menopause are prescribed two measures daily, although younger women may be given more. The gel is rubbed into the underside of the arms or the legs or the lower body. It takes about five minutes to dry and the area must not be washed or have any other lotions applied to it for an hour. A template is provided to illustrate the area to be coated as the amount absorbed can be affected by the size of the area and how well the gel is rubbed in.

Advantages
- The gel is easy to use – the delivery is physiological.
- There is no skin irritation or unsightly patches.

Disadvantages
- The gel can be messy and needs to dry (although our medical advisor's patients like it).
- It can be difficult to use before going to bed for women with partners as skin contact needs to be avoided for an hour in case it is absorbed by another person. It is best done after a shower and allowed to dry whilst putting on make-up.

CRINONE

As well as oestrogen gels there is a vaginal natural progesterone gel called Crinone. (This should not be confused with natural progesterone cream, most commonly brand-named Progest, and sold as a complementary therapy. Research has shown there may be dangers in mistakenly assuming that this can be used as the progestogen element of conventional oestrogen HRT – more details in Chapter 6). Crinone is absorbed systemically (i.e. absorbed throughout the body and affecting the whole system) and can therefore be used as the progesterone element of oestrogen-only HRT. It's used with an applicator and women need to make six applications over 12 progesterone days.

The advantage of Crinone is that there are fewer side-effects than when taking progestogens orally. Some women, of course, suffer them more than others, but this form of progesterone is a more physiological method of absorption than any of those discussed earlier. The disadvantage is that it can be messy and if the bleed comes early – within the 12 days that the gel is being applied – it has to be continued. Very messy indeed! There are pessaries available which will do the same job.

Vaginal HRT

This is helpful for women who cannot tolerate or who don't want to take HRT. The oestrogen can be applied to the vagina for local relief of symptoms if vaginal dryness or frequent cystitis are found to be a problem. It can be used as an add-on to full-scale HRT if additional help is needed for these symptoms.

Vaginal HRT is available in cream, pessary, vaginal tablet and vaginal ring form – the latter is designed to release oestradiol over three months. There are some natural oestrogen and some synthetic oestrogen preparations.

Initially, it's advised that the creams or pessaries be used frequently and then reduced as the oestrogen is believed to be more readily absorbed once the vaginal lining begins to change. If these preparations are used long-term or if they contain synthetic oestrogens, they can be absorbed systemically into the blood stream and a progestogen may sometimes be needed in addition.

Advantages
- It can be useful for local symptoms and for women who cannot tolerate systemic HRT.
- This form of HRT produces fewer of the risks and side-effects.

Disadvantages
- It can be messy.
- It can damage latex on condoms and should not be used as a lubricant during sex as the hormone can be absorbed by a partner.
- It doesn't have the overall benefits of systemic HRT.

NASAL SPRAY

A method of delivering oestrogen that is currently being developed is a nasal spray which would involve a squirt in each nostril twice a day. In a clinical trial completed in June 1999 involving 420 women, the oestradiol spray was found to be as effective in relieving symptoms of the menopause as tablets, but without the side-effects associated with either pills or patches. In women who have not had a hysterectomy, it would have to be opposed by progesterone in some other form. It will be available in the UK from May 2001.

INTER-UTERINE SYSTEM (IUS)

A new development is the Mirena, a T-shaped inter-uterine system (IUS) that slowly releases the progestogen, levonorgestrel. It is made of a light plastic material and the stem of the T is a bit thicker than the rest. This stem contains a tiny storage system of levonorgestrel which thins the lining of the womb. After insertion it is effective for five years.

Mirena is licensed as a contraceptive, but there is growing experience of the IUS for women who require the progesterone element of HRT. It can be combined with oestrogen implants, tablets or patches, making it another form of continuous combined 'no-bleed' HRT. Because the hormone is delivered directly to the lining of the uterus, the dose of progestogen is less and therefore is found to cause fewer side-effects.

The real bonus is its effectiveness as a contraceptive. Mirena can be used during the perimenopause to deal with heavy and erratic periods and to counter the risk of pregnancy. It is also the only way of achieving a 'no-bleed' regimen for the perimenopausal woman.

The use of Mirena as an HRT is not yet licensed in the UK, although it can be prescribed under the care of a gynaecologist. The novelist, Rosie Thomas – you may remember from Chapter 1 – was given it after her Himalayan haemorrhage and has had no more problems and no further menopausal symptoms. In a number of other countries the IUS is licensed for use as an HRT and Dr Marion Everitt who runs the NHS Menopause Clinic in Leeds believes it wil be licensed in the UK within the next three years.

As mentioned earlier, Everitt is a great supporter of the Mirena, going so far as to describe it as 'the best thing since the pill for women's health'. Where it's been used in hospitals for the treatment of heavy periods the rate of hysterectomy has been halved. As a remedy for other menopausal symptoms, she is not convinced of the usefulness of progesterone on its own, but says Mirena is excellent in opposition to all forms of oestrogen-only doses. It has, in her clinical experience, no systemic side-effects – no bloating, heaviness, premenstrual pain or mood swings.

In her own case, when she began having flushes and night sweats at the age of 45 she did nothing for a year as the symptoms were not debilitating. Then it got worse. Hot sweats became embarrassing in meetings because perspiration would pour down her face. She became irritable and suffered from poor memory and concentration and decided that she must find something to suit her. There was, she thought, no point in struggling with these difficulties. She couldn't get the patch to stay on, three different types of tablet gave her headaches and she finally hit upon oestrogene gel and the Mirena and hasn't looked back. 'Brilliant!', she says.

She did for herself what she tries to do for all her patients. She uses blood tests to help with diagnosis and tailors treatment to the individual through trial and error. She reckons to have a 70 per cent success rate in the clinic of women who feel marvellous. The other 30 per cent, she says, are probably disappointed because they overestimated what HRT could do for them. It will never, she points out, make you quite as good as you were and we shouldn't rely on it to make us look younger, just to keep us active and healthy.

She does recommend, if there is no GP who specialises in menopause at your practice, that you try to attend a specialist clinic. Too often, she says, GPs stick with the pre-packed formulations and are not so willing to 'fiddle around'. She has been known to prescribe the oestrogen part of one pack of pills and the progestogen of another or to combine Mirena with oestrogen pills. GPs, of course, often have neither the knowledge nor the time to devote to this kind of patient-centred treatment, but it seems essential if you are to find the right form of HRT for you.

COST OF HRT PRESCRIPTIONS

The Labour MP Dr Howard Stoate attempted to bring a Private Member's Bill before Parliament in the autumn of 1999, highlighting the unfair charges for HRT prescriptions. If the oestrogen and progesterone is combined in the same pill, as in continuous combined HRT, there is only one prescription charge for the preparation. If your doctor has the generosity to prescribe for six months on one 'scrip, you pay only £6, but double, £12, if you're on sequential combined pills or combined patches. You pay for each drug because the NHS argues that even though the tablets are necessary for your treatment and come in one pack, they are two separate drugs in individual tablets – oestrogen and progestogen.

Then, if the doctor prescribes only one month's supply of pills at a time, as some do, and you're on sequential HRT, you could end up with an annual bill of £144. There is no progress yet on changing the charging regime, but it's worth talking to your doctor about extending the duration of the supply on each prescription once you are happy with your treatment. If that doesn't work, or if you take drugs for any other condition – asthma, for example – it is worth getting a pre-paid prescription certificate from your health authority. It currently costs £86.20 for a whole year and covers everything you have on prescription.

OTHER TREATMENTS

Below are some less commonly offered forms of possible treatment which do not come under the category of conventional HRT.

TIBOLONE (BRAND NAME LIVIAL)

This is a treatment that has been around for some 15 years. It is not classified as hormone replacement therapy because it's a synthetic compound which has the combined action of oestrogens and progestogens and is known as 'gonadomimetic'. Tibolone acts on the hormone receptors, but does not stimulate the lining of the womb, so it is a bleed-free treatment. It can treat menopausal symptoms and it is licensed to prevent osteoporosis, although its role in the possible prevention of heart disease is unclear. For women who are worried about endometriosis it can be useful as it doesn't stimulate the lining of the womb. It also acts on the androgen receptors, so it can help with testosterone levels and consequently can help to increase libido.

Tibolone is best suited to older, post-menopausal women. If it is used within the year after the last period it can cause irregular bleeding. It may also have androgenic side-effects, including unwanted hair growth and acne. Women who don't like the idea of taking a synthetic drug may not want to take it.

RALOXIFENE (BRAND NAME EVISTA)

Raloxifene, a 'designer oestrogen', is said to be an exciting new development in the treatment of women at risk from post-menopausal osteoporosis. It is a selective oestrogen receptor modulator (SERM), and is related to the anti-breast cancer drug, Tamoxifen.

SERMs are a new class of drugs that work selectively in oestrogen-sensitive tissues. They mimic the action of oestrogen on certain body tissues, such as bone, and so have some of the benefits of oestrogen without the unwanted side-effects.

Raloxifene acts like oestrogen on the bone and studies have shown that it has a good effect in raising bone density in the spine and the hip and in lowering fracture risk in the spine of both apparently healthy women and of women already suffering from osteoporosis. It has no effect on the womb and so is not associated in any way with the monthly cycle.

Recent research has shown a reduced risk of breast cancer in women using the drug compared with women taking a placebo. Further work is being carried out on the claims that it can help to prevent heart disease. It does reduce cholesterol levels. Dr Jane Somerville, Emeritus Professor of Cardiology at the Imperial College School of Medicine in London is concerned about the most recent research carried out in America, led by Nanette Wenger showing slightly negative results with a small rise in thrombosis, similar to that in conventional HRT, in women taking the drug. Dr Somerville is worried that the trials may have been stopped too early and may not have come to the correct conclusion.

The irony of this 'designer' oestrogen is that it has no role in treating the symptoms for which women most frequently seek HRT, in fact it has been shown to worsen hot flushes. In future SERMs may be developed that will deal with all the problems associated with menopause, but none is on the horizon as yet. Experts predict that women may be offered conventional HRT to deal with menopausal symptoms and then SERMs as preventative treatment for osteoporosis once the hot-flush stage has passed. It is, though, an experimental option and it will be some time before solid data is available on long-term risks and benefits.

TESTOSTERONE HRT

As we've already discussed, testosterone, usually seen as a male hormone, is produced by women too, albeit at lower levels than in most men. It is produced in the ovaries and adrenal glands and is believed to be a vital female sex hormone, affecting libido. Research suggests that one in three menopausal women suffers from low libido, or a lack of interest in sex. There could, of course, be a number of factors influencing this, such as the quality of a relationship or other illnessess. Some of us may be pefectly content with a slowing down of sexual activity. If it is a problem for you – and it is apparently especially common in women who have had hysterectomy with oophorectomy (removal of the womb and ovaries) – it may be worth trying testosterone replacement.

Research carried out in the USA and published in September 2000 showed that some women might benefit from the therapy. Studies began in a number of cities around Britain in August 2000 to test the efficacy of the testosterone patch, so the treatment is very much in the experimental stage. It is already acknowledged that there may be unwanted side-effects such as the deepening of the voice and male-pattern hair growth.

WHEN HRT IS NOT SUITABLE

Absolute contra-indications are as follows:

- Active thrombosis.
- An undiagnosed breast mass.
- Active breast or endometrial cancer. Women who have had these cancers in the past may be able to take HRT, but should discuss it with their doctor. Several random trials of the use of HRT in women with breast cancer are currently in progress or are planned. The available limited data on the use of HRT in patients who have had endometrial cancer shows little evidence of any further detrimental effect in terms of recurrence. One random trial is currently under way.
- Acute liver disease. This is obviously a problem with oral HRT as it has to pass through the liver, but if menopausal symptoms are severe it may be possible to take HRT by a non-oral route under the supervision of a specialist.
- Undiagnosed vaginal bleeding (the causes need to be investigated).
- Pregnancy or breastfeeding.

HRT should be used with caution in the following cases:

- A strong family history of breast cancer.
- A strong family history of thrombo-embolism (blood clots in the legs or lungs).
- A previous history of benign breast lumps.

- A previous history of gallstones, as HRT may stimulate them. It is recommended that women who have already had gallstones, but have not had their gall bladder removed, use a non-oral method if they chose HRT.
- Any previous liver disease, even if mild. Again, a non-oral method would be recommended and liver function would need to be monitored.
- Migraines can be made worse by HRT but, confusingly, in some cases can be improved!
- Heart disease.
- Obesity.
- Endometriosis can in some cases be reactivated by oestrogen therapy. If this is the case, Tibolone may be prescribed. Any symptoms should be reported to a doctor immediately.
- Fibroids can also be stimulated by oestrogen albeit rarely unless, of course, you have had a hysterectomy. Regular pelvic examinations are recommended and any symptoms, such as bleeding, should be reported.
- Epilepsy might be made worse by HRT and some anti-epileptic drugs will mean the required dose of HRT should be increased. It's best given by patch or gel to avoid a dangerous interaction with anti-convulsant medication.
- Multiple sclerosis may very rarely be worsened by HRT.
- Rarer conditions such as porphyria, some kidney and heart problems and Roter Syndrome may have reactions to HRT. It's better to discuss any chronic disorder with a doctor before deciding whether or not to take HRT.
- High blood pressure does not mean HRT has to be excluded. Natural oestrogens have not been shown to raise blood pressure further in the majority of women; in fact in some cases they have had the effect of lowering it. A small percentage of women have been shown to develop a sensitivity to some forms of HRT, particularly those using equine oestrogens, and the blood

pressure has gone up. Even these women should be able to take in some form of HRT.

- Diabetes has not been shown to be affected by HRT as long as it is well controlled. Close checks should be made on blood sugar levels at the start of the treatment.
- Otosclerosis – an inherited cause of hearing loss – can become much worse during pregnancy, suggesting a hormonal link. Specialist advice is needed before embarking on HRT.
- Varicose veins should not be of concern unless they are very bad, in which case it may be better not to take HRT. It should be stopped if the veins become painful or inflamed. (Joan Bakewell had hers 'stripped out' in her mid-thirties – the only cosmetic surgery she has ever considered – and went on to take HRT successfully for more than 20 years.)

If you are taking any other medication, for example for asthma, epilepsy or thyroid problems, you should, of course, discuss these with a doctor. Everyone should be given a thorough check-up, including medical history, before embarking on HRT. Dr Marion Everitt from the Leeds Menopause Clinic is in favour of the full MOT before prescribing HRT. Blood tests, a pelvic exam and, in her view, a mammogram give a picture of the state of health before HRT and are helpful in the regular necessary monitoring which should continue during treatment.

WHEN TO START TAKING HRT

Obviously, you don't have to wait until after the menopause to begin. Once the perimenopausal symptoms we've already discussed have begun and are giving you grief you can start selecting your type of HRT depending on whether or not your periods have stopped. Women who had an artificial menopause by having their

ovaries removed or a medical menopause as a result of radiotherapy
are advised to start immediately.

The Amarant Trust advises starting to take HRT if the
menopausal symptoms begin to impinge on your life, not necessarily
at the first sign of a hot flush. Past the menopause, you can take HRT
for its long-term benefits – but only if you decide you want to in
either case, having weighed up all the pros and cons (see Chapter 5).

HRT AND CONTRACEPTION

Mirena works as a contraceptive, but none of the other methods of
hormone replacement do. You need to think about what type of
contraception to use during the perimenopause and it's
recommended for up to two years after the menopause, just to be
certain. You may still be taking the pill, as Penny Heeley did until
she was 50–52. Her doctor then suggested she might like to come
off it and she has not had a period since. Do use another form of
contraception whilst coming off the pill until you are certain you
are post-menopausal, as even though fertility declines with age, it
is still possible to have a surprise, as Cherie Blair found.

HRT DOSAGE

Most types of HRT come in different strengths to suit the
individual's body chemistry. Basically, we need enough oestrogen
to control minor menopausal symptoms with minimal side-effects,
although women with more severe symptoms such as bad hot
flushes may require higher doses of oestrogen. As we get older and
the symptoms decrease doses may be lowered.

The recommended daily doses of oestrogen for protection
against bone loss are:

0.625mg conjugated oestrogens in daily tablets

   or 2mg of oestradiol

   or 1.5mg piperazine oestrone sulphate

   or 50mcg of oestradiol in once- or twice-weekly patches

1.5mg of oestradiol in gel form daily

50mg oestradiol in implant form

2.5mg daily tibolone.

The most recent evidence, however, shows that in older women bone protection can be achieved with the lower dose continuous combined 'no-bleed' HRTs.

Doctors will recommend the necessary levels of progestogens to eradicate the risk of endometrial cancer in balance with the dose of oestrogen.

There have been some horror stories about HRT-prescribing among the women I have talked to. One interviewee saw three different doctors in trying to get the right HRT. The first told her, 'It's a must, think of your bones.' And gave her Prempak C. It made her feel unwell and depressed, although she finds it difficult, in retrospect, to distinguish between what was chemically induced and what was normal for her situation. The second doctor was wholly intent on eradicating her symptoms and prescribed a continuous combined HRT Premique. She didn't get on with that either – it gave her stomach problems – and when she went to a third doctor he asked when she'd had her last period. When it was finally established that she was peri-, not post-menopausal he told her she shouldn't have been on what she was given as it was a 'no-bleed' HRT, designed for post-menopausal women. This third one was reluctant to prescribe at all, saying, 'Our mothers didn't have it,' but she was insistent and finally hit upon a brand which suited her.

It's easy to blame GPs – and, as I pointed out earlier, doctors carry as much cultural baggage about what it means to be a menopausal woman as any of us – but we should bear in mind, as I've said, that HRT and its relationship with the endocrine system is a phenomenally complex subject which needs a great deal of study to comprehend fully. As Dr Everitt has pointed out, GPs often lack knowledge, time – and, in some cases, the inclination – to see each woman and her body chemistry as unique. You may be lucky and hit on a pre-packaged formulation which suits you perfectly. If not, there's no need to give up.

With the information in this book, advice from organisations like the Amarant Trust or, best of all, access to a specialist menopause clinic, it should be possible, perhaps using a variety of methods, to find a form of HRT which is right for you. The next generation of women most probably won't have this problem as researchers at the forefront of the field believe that in 10 to 20 years' time there will be sophisticated tests to establish what you need and to give doctors the information from which to tailor the perfect supplement for you. Until then, don't be fobbed off by ignorance, reluctance or, indeed, misplaced over-enthusiasm, in your GP. (See Useful Addresses for The Amarant Trust's HRT compendium of current treatments and prices and The King's Regimen, designed to help prescribers to tailor an HRT to an individual patient's needs.)

WHEN TO STOP TAKING HRT

If you feel well on HRT there is no reason to stop taking it at all. Dr Marion Everitt, who firmly believes menopause to be a deficiency disease, is content for women to stay on it for ever, in much the same way as a diabetic would take insulin for the rest of her life. If you are taking HRT to prevent osteoporosis there is new evidence that bone loss begins again one year after the treatment has ended, so again, you may want to consider continuing for ever if you are at high risk of bone disease. Teresa Gorman has taken it for more than 20 years, as has Joan Bakewell. Joan Jenkins, founder president of the charity Women's Health, has taken it for more than 25 years. None of them intends to stop, as they feel so well on it.

There were worries in the early 1990s about addiction. A gynaecologist, Dr Susan Bewley, published an article in the *Lancet* expressing concern that some women might become dependent on HRT. Her paper argues that oestrogens have powerful psychoactive effects, which means they can lift the mood. The papers blew the story up, claiming that HRT was as addictive as heroin. In fact, Dr Bewley was merely warning about the possibility of dependency (and Joan Bakewell and Jo Wagerman's stories of feeling ghastly when they stopped would bear out that it is possible to depend on it for well-being); but her main concern was with implants where tachyphylaxis and overdosing, as discussed earlier, are a risk.

Bewley's warnings do indicate that care needs to be taken when coming off HRT. An abrupt stop can lead to the return of the same symptoms you had before as, effectively, you are putting your body through another menopause, suddenly depriving it of hormones. If you are taking tablets you can reduce the dose gradually over two or three months with the help of your doctor. You should be prescribed a lower dose of oestrogen and then after several weeks increase the time lapse between each dose. So, instead of taking a tablet every day, take one every other day, then every four days and so on. The dose in a patch can be reduced and then you can tail it off by cutting the patches into smaller pieces as Lesley Hilton did. If you have implants, reduce the dose every six months for a year or so, then stop altogether. Progestogen should be taken until there is no further bleeding to account for any residual oestrogen left in the body. This can take two to three years, so implants should only be embarked upon when you are absolutely sure HRT is for you as it is a long-term commitment.

But don't make that commitment until you have considered both the long-term risks and benefits of HRT . . .

CHAPTER 5

THE PROS AND CONS
OF HRT

As I was researching these chapters and talking to all my friends and acquaintances – even women I bumped into in the supermarket queue – about their menopause, one close pal sent me a leaflet through the post which she had picked up at her doctor's surgery. *Health Facts Every Post-Menopausal Woman Should Know* trotted out the usual scary stuff about 'one in five women die of coronary heart disease, one in 12 women will develop breast cancer and 50 per cent of all women are at risk of osteoporosis' (somewhat exaggerated claims, as pointed out in earlier chapters). Others sent me more 'information' leaflets for HRT, which stated categorically that HRT can prevent heart disease and osteoporosis. Most of them were found in hospitals, health centres or shops and the small print at the back often showed they were financed by leading drug companies that make profits from the sale of HRT. This chapter is based on the best and most recent work we've been able to uncover.

WHAT HRT CAN DO

The potential beneficial effects of HRT on the wide-ranging symptoms of the menopause are as follows:

HOT FLUSHES AND NIGHT SWEATS

These have been shown to clear dramatically within days or weeks of starting HRT. This often leads, as many of my own sample have reported, to better sleep patterns which in turn reduce insomnia, tiredness and irritability.

VAGINAL DRYNESS AND URINARY PROBLEMS

HRT can reduce vaginal dryness and the thinning of the vaginal lining whether taken orally, in the form of patches or locally applied cream. Women whose only symptom is vaginal dryness are advised to try an oestrogen cream in the first instance as it generally does not need to be opposed by progesterone. Women who take low-dose HRT in other forms, but still have the problem, may find it helpful to use a cream as well.

There is, though, as I have suggested earlier, an important question to ask about vaginal dryness. Dr Hilary Jones says that doctors are often puzzled by complaints about vaginal dryness because there seems to be little correlation between the reported symptom and the physical state of the vagina. Some women have symptoms with very little change visible on examination, whereas other women have no symptoms of dryness when fairly obvious physical changes have occurred. This would seem to bear out my own common-sense theory that vaginal dryness probably depends more on the head than the 'down below'. An attentive, attractive and exciting lover will probably get things moving better than any creams and potions. It's also known that regular intercourse can stimulate the vagina.

As a journalist with a special interest in these issues I've had lots of letters in my time from women in middle age who are desperate that they no longer get 'turned on' by their husbands and fear that he may be straying because of their lack of interest. I've also had a number of letters, some months or even years later, from those same women. Some of them say they were left by those erring husbands and almost immediately found a new lover and things improved. The novelist Rosie Thomas and Vera Ivers from the Older Women's Network both reported this to me. Others, who had also been dumped, found huge release once they'd got over the shock and grief. They enjoyed being free from a critical, middle-aged misery guts and got on and did their own thing, whether it involved a sexual relationship or not. Others decided in the long term that their marriage had other qualities – shared history, family and interests – that made it worth working for. Hanging in and talking things over often resolved the physical side of the relationship. If you're feeling miserable because of lack of attention, don't blame yourself or your hormones, look for other solutions first.

Oestrogen can help to reduce the feeling of needing to empty the bladder frequently and urgently. Recurrent urinary infections may be prevented as HRT reduces vaginal acidity, but there is disagreement as to what dose and duration of treatment makes a difference. It may take a year for vaginal and urinary symptoms to respond to HRT. Stress incontinence needs extra help. There are drugs available for unstable bladders, as discussed in Chapter 3, and surgery for stress incontinence, but exercise is the first line of attack. Go for that pelvic floor!

SKIN AND HAIR

Teresa Gorman tells me she can visit an old people's home and tell at a glance which women are HRT-users and which are not by the quality of their skin and hair. From her own point of view she says HRT has given her 'plumptitude'. The skin all over her body, she says, is in amazingly good nick and even when she dieted and lost weight a few years ago her skin shrank with her because it is still elastic. This she puts down to the effects of oestrogen on the collagen which supports the skin. She also says her hair has not thinned and her gums have not receded (she's 67).

The most recent research seems to support her contention. The skin begins to thin quite rapidly from the age of 40, due to ageing, but HRT does seem to slow the process because it has been shown to help to maintain collagen. The hair, too, can thicken and improve its condition during treatment. Edwina Currie has found this to be the case, although in her case the moisture content of both her skin and hair has not been helped. She needs lots of moisturisers and conditioner.

In some cases, HRT has been shown to increase the water content of the skin, as well as improving its blood flow. It's said that this can help a dry throat and mouth and burning eyes.

A joint German and Chilean study, reported in the Lancet in 1999, showed that a group of women tested by university gynaecologists in both countries demonstrated that those with higher oestrogen levels had younger-looking skin. A big American study, published in 1997, and carried out by Dr Laura Dunn at the University of California tested some 4000 post-menopausal women between the ages of 40 and 74. Cases of dry and wrinkled skin were 25 per cent to 30 per cent fewer in women who had used oestrogen compared with those who hadn't.

There is a rider to this research, though. Dunn also reported that, once wrinkles set in, some women became so depressed about it that they began to take less care of themselves. The ones whose skin didn't dry or wrinkle excessively may simply have been slapping on more moisture and taking more care with diet and exercise. (Personally, I think being a bit overweight is a great help in all this. There's nothing like a bit of fat under the skin to fill out the crinkles! This could also be influenced by the fact that fatter women tend to produce more of their own oestrogen.)

DEPRESSION AND MOOD SWINGS

A number of bodies, including the North American Menopause Society, say there is no link between the menopause and depression, although, anecdotally, lots of women, including myself, say they have experienced an improvement in psychological well-being after taking HRT. Some studies show that mood swings and depression improve with HRT; others don't, and there is controversy about what might bring about improvement where it exists. The British Menopause Society say there are lots of factors to consider, including:

- **The placebo effect**
  Women with menopausal symptoms value an explanation of why they are feeling unwell and this alone may produce considerable psychological benefit. Double blind placebo controlled trials have shown this to be the case.
- **The domino effect**
  Removing hot flushes and night sweats with HRT can improve women's sleeping patterns and, consequently, their mood. It has been found that women who have not had these symptoms are less likely to improve psychologically with HRT.
- **The aphrodisiac effect**
  If vaginal dryness is relieved by HRT, some women will experience improved libido, but the Society's conclusions seem to tally with my own: 'Mostly, however, it is the quality of the relationship and the health, interest and potency of the male partner that is more important in achieving a good sex life.'

MEMORY LOSS

A lot of women describe a kind of brain scrambling effect as they become perimenopausal – you may remember Moyra Livesey of the Rylstone WI saying she couldn't even remember the names of her close friends at WI meetings. The mechanisms of the action of oestrogen on brain function are not entirely clear, but it is believed to act on neural growth and to improve blood flow to the brain.

Studies carried out at Yale University in the United States tested women's performance in certain memory functions, such as remembering telephone numbers. They used magnetic resonance imaging (MRI), a process which detects differences in the magnetic properties between oxygenated and deoxygenated blood. By this technique, blood flow and oxygen concentration levels in brain regions can be detected. The results showed that in women who were taking oestrogen the brain activation patterns were similar to those normally seen in younger women. The study went on for 21 days and although there was no actual improvement of memory performance during the period of study, the researchers believe the brain activation changes would eventually lead to improvements. Their findings were similar to those in two other US studies carried out by the Laboratory of Personality and Cognition and the National Institute of Ageing.

In August 2000, the *Lancet* published the results of research carried out by Kristine Yaffe and colleagues at the University of California who measured the level of oestradiol in 425 women over the age of 65. Their cognitive peformance was assessed when the study began, between 1986 and 1988, and again six years later. All the women showed a slight decline in cognitive function, but among those with the lowest natural levels of oestradiol, 16 per cent (17 out of 106) showed a significant decline six years later. For those with the highest levels, only five per cent (5 out of 94) showed a similiar decline.

ALZHEIMER'S DISEASE

These research projects have an obvious implication in the understanding of Alzheimer's Disease and in January 2000 the

Medical Research Council in Britain announced that it was funding an extra branch of the WISDOM (Women's International Study of Long Duration Oestrogen After Menopause) trials which would look further into whether HRT can reduce cognitive decline and dementia in older women.

Dr Eef Hogervorst from the Oxford project to Investigate Memory and Ageing confirms that oestrogen can enhance neurotransmitters, cerebral blood flow and improve the function of the cells. Oestrogen also has vascular effects on the blood pressure and its flow around the body and this may have an effect on Alzheimer's.

She is doubtful that the fall in oestrogen at the time of the menopause is of real significance in the 'brain-scrambling' symptoms, as it is reported by a relatively small number of women, and men have larger cognitive dips with age than do women. In her experience, when oestrogen is measured, some women reporting memory problems still have high levels of oestrogen and vice versa. She believes it is more likely that cognitive problems, like emotional problems, may be due to other life stresses.

Hogervorst explains that, where HRT has been shown to improve memory, no allowance was made for socio-economic class, so improvements may be because of the 'healthy user effect'. In other words, women taking HRT may be better educated, more concerned about their health and have a healthier diet and lifestyle. Truly random studies are hard to do, she says, because women are likely to know whether or not they have been given hormones.

In studies where HRT appears to have protected women against Alzheimer's Disease the healthy user effect may again be a factor and there is no evidence that HRT will help women who already have Alzheimer's Disease. In fact, women treated with Premarin were found to have actually got worse. There will be more conclusive answers on whether HRT improves memory and protects against Alzheimer's Disease when the results of the WISDOM trial are published in 2006, so newspaper headlines which in recent years have proclaimed 'Women on HRT stay clever and alert for longer' and ' HRT could aid memory after menopause' appear a little premature.

PARKINSON'S DISEASE

In November 1998, the Fifth International Congress of Parkinson's Disease and Movement Disorders heard that 202 women had been involved in a 15-year study at the Mayo Clinic in the USA, and the results of the study showed that those who developed Parkinson's Disease tended not to have used HRT. A link between oestrogen deficiency and Parkinson's Disease was also suggested by the observation that women who had had a hysterectomy had a threefold risk of contracting Parkinson's compared with those who had not. This research comes as no comfort to my mother, who took HRT for nearly 25 years and developed Parkinson's Disease in her early seventies.

OSTEOPOROSIS

Bone is renewed in our bodies throughout our lives. Bone is lost because the replacing bone cells (osteoblasts) don't keep up with the excavating cells (osteoclasts). When we are young, the rate of bone formation exceeds bone loss and then it levels out in adulthood. From 35 to 40, the rate at which worn-out bone is replaced by bone-building cells slows, so bone density decreases. Whether this becomes a problem will depend on a number of factors, such as how much bone has been built up in the first place, diet and exercise. Smoking is thought to increase the risk of osteoporosis by up to 400 per cent.

The age-related decline is a greater problem for women than men because we tend to build up less bone in the first place and we live longer, but the effects of natural menopause and living longer do need to be kept in perspective. Data on fracture rates in different countries would suggest that genetic differences and lifestyle are more important than whether one is a woman or a man. It's thought that a poorer-quality lifestyle (in terms of diet and exercise) rather than longevity is the main reason for a three-fold increase in the rate of fracture among women over the last 30 years in Europe. Nevertheless, the number of osteoporotic fractures is expected to rise again in the next few years because we are living longer. In Western Europe, the number of fractures is expected to at least double in the next 50 years.

At the time of the menopause there is accelerated bone loss, thought to be caused by lack of oestrogen. The precise mechanism by which oestrogen affects bone is unclear, but it is thought to decrease the rate of bone turnover. HRT replaces the role of oestrogen and therefore helps to reduce bone loss. It also helps to strengthen the existing bone structure and can have a positive building effect on bone mass in the initial stages of treatment – the degree of improvement will depend on the dose. The details of this were explained in Chapter 4 and it is still unclear how low the dose can be to achieve the desired effect. Some progestogens (the c-19 variety) may add to the effect of oestrogen. Depending on the dose and the individual, the rate of bone loss will plateau out or continue, but at a slower rate. The real benefits are gained with long-term use of HRT. It is thought that the risk of hip fracture is reduced by about 30 per cent and spinal fracture by 50 per cent when treatment is undertaken for five years. Continuing to take HRT for ten years is calculated to reduce density loss by 10 per cent to 15 per cent which would otherwise result in a doubling of the fracture risk. Some specialists say that for women already suffering from osteoporosis the positive effects are even more marked.

However, as Juliet Compston, reader in metabolic bone disease and an honorary consultant physician at the University of Cambridge School of Clinical Medicine, points out, the issue of whether HRT reduces hip fractures is very controversial. All the evidence comes from observational studies which are subject to bias and likely to overestimate the benefits of HRT, because women who choose to take HRT are, for social and economic reasons, generally healthier in the first place than those who do not.

Crucially, the reported positive benefits of HRT for the prevention and treatment of post-menopausal osteoporosis will only be gained as long as you carry on taking it. These effects decline rapidly after treatment stops so, to decrease the risk of hip fracture, HRT would have to be given to women in their sixties and seventies. The problem is that women usually begin taking HRT during or immediately after the menopause and then stop after a few years, whereas most osteoporotic fractures occur after the age of 65. Long-term use is necessary to have any substantial impact on the incidence of fractures. There is no evidence that taking HRT at an early age delays the average age of fracture.

After HRT is stopped, bone loss resumes within a year and bone turnover decreases to the level of untreated women within three to six months, which probably accounts for the lack of fracture protection in past users. But because HRT needs to be taken long term, the benefits have to be balanced with the risks of long-term use. For this reason, women who are post-menopausal and have concerns about osteoporosis, but are also worried about the associated breast cancer risk, say, may want to consider the new designer HRT, raloxifene. As mentioned in Chapter 4 (p. 133), it has no role in the suppression of hot flushes and night sweats, but is useful for osteoporosis prevention once these symptoms have passed.

Teeth

Loss of bone density associated with osteoporosis may contribute to tooth loss and peridontal disease, so there is a suggestion that HRT taken for osteoporosis may also have a beneficial effect on oral health.

MUSCLE STRENGTH

Research carried out by Professor Roger Woledge at the Royal Orthopaedic Hospital in Stanmore, north London, hit the headlines in May 1999 – 'HRT treatment can even make it easier to do the gardening'. The team of researchers studied more than 100 middle-aged and elderly women, half of whom were taking HRT, and measured the strength and size of their muscles and the density of the bones. The women were asked to perform simple tasks such as squeezing a specially designed metal bar which monitored their strength and mimicked everyday actions such as opening door-knobs or screw-top jars. Researchers found that muscle strength in the HRT group was up to 30 per cent greater (average 15 per cent) than among the others, although there was no significant difference in muscle size between the two groups.

There is ample anecdotal evidence that for those women who can take HRT (in Professor Woledge's trial, 12 women dropped out in the early stages because of short-term side-effects of the drug), the treatment is useful in boosting strength and energy. Janet Paraskeva, who, at 54, took on the difficult job of running the Law Society after heading the National Lottery Charities Board since its inception, began taking HRT when she was 51 and was finding menopausal symptoms a trial. Hot flushes were a bore in meetings, but her greatest concern was feeling tired all the time and lacking her usual 'oomph'. A number of friends had told her HRT was 'good stuff'. It had given them bags of energy and made them feel rejuvenated. It has made her feel stronger and fitter.

HEART DISEASE

Just as virtually every drug company leaflet (and most books on the subject) will tell you HRT will prevent osteoporosis, without adding any of the riders outlined above, so, too, they will proclaim HRT is good for the heart. Not necessarily so. HRT and its link with coronary heart disease (CHD) is one of the big controversies that are awaiting new evidence from a number of current long-term studies before anyone can accurately pronounce on whether it is helpful or harmful.

Coronary heart disease is, as outlined in earlier chapters, the primary cause of death among post-menopausal women and it has always been claimed that women's risk of heart disease rises significantly after the menopause, whereas the rise for men in their fifties and sixties has been a steady progression. In *The Healthy Heart Handbook for Women*, Dr David Ashton disputes this received wisdom, and goes as far as to say that this contention, promulgated by the media, the women's magazines and the pharmaceutical industry, is wrong. Ashton calls any connection made between menopause and heart disease 'a myth'. He shows there is no sudden increase in heart-disease rates after the menopause and demonstrates, on the contrary, that the rate of increase in women aged 30 to 34 through to 60 to 64 years is almost the same. He acknowledges that the number of heart attacks in women goes up after the age of 50, but says it is a steady rise, not a sudden leap, and is due to the continuing effects of ageing, not the menopause.

The reason, he says, why death rates in men and women are similar in older age groups is not because rates increase in women, but because they fall slightly in men, probably because risk factors such as stress at work, unhealthy business lunches, heavy drinking, smoking and lack of exercise are less prevalent as men get older and take things easier (a lesson here for us, perhaps). These more accurate conclusions about men and women are now beginning to come through as medical researchers have shifted their earlier bias towards testing their hypotheses and treatments in this field solely on the male.

Nevertheless, it is still frequently categorically stated that taking HRT can reduce your risk of heart disease by up to 50 per cent. This claim has been made as a result of the following findings:

- There is an increased risk of heart disease (double) in women who have had ovaries removed before the menopause, but less risk if they have oestrogen therapy afterwards.
- Studies observing women on HRT appear to show a lower risk. For example, a large study in the USA followed the health of more than 120,000 nurses from 1976 onwards. By 1986 almost 50,000 of them had passed through the menopause and about half of them had taken HRT. In those taking the treatment, the rate of death from heart disease was 39 per cent less than in non-takers and the amount of coronary artery disease was 49 per cent less than in non-users. In an overview of 25 studies reported by mid-1997 it was found that the relative risk of CHD for women using oestrogen therapy was 40 per cent less than in those who had never used it. Relative risk with use of oestrogen together with progestogen was similar.
- There is evidence that oestrogen in the body can have a positive effect on blood constituents and reduce bad (LDL) cholesterol and increase good (HDL) cholesterol. There is also evidence that oestrogen can dilate blood vessels. Increasing the amount of blood that can flow through can counteract the narrowing effect of fatty deposits in the blood vessels.
- It has been suggested that progestogens also play a part in keeping the heart healthy by preventing the proliferation of smooth muscle cells that line blood vessels, and the formation of fatty deposits within them, which can in turn cause heart attacks or strokes. On the other hand, whilst oestrogen can reduce the tendency of the blood to clot, progestogens tend to have the opposite effect, although it is believed that the doses used in modern HRT are probably too small to have serious ill-effects.

Still, it seems to be becoming more generally accepted that there are difficulties in establishing an actual cause and effect relationship between menopause, HRT and coronary heart disease. There are problems, for instance, with the oestrogen and cholesterol connection. Although it seems to suggest that oestrogen indirectly reduces the 'furring up of arteries' it is now known that lowering cholesterol levels affords only about 30 per cent of the protective effect against heart disease, so only a third of the reported reduction in risk can be laid at the door of the effect of oestrogen on cholesterol levels. This 30 per cent may, of course, be extremely useful in reducing dangerous cholesterol levels just enough for those women whose levels are exceptionally high.

It should also be pointed out that it is the liver which produces 80 per cent of the body's cholesterol, so HRT in tablet form, where the hormones have to make the 'first pass' through the liver (generally associated with unpleasant side-effects), may in fact be more useful in relation to CHD than other forms of delivery. The contention that oestrogen can dilate blood vessels is based on experimental work and this too is questionable. There is no evidence to show that the effects shown in experiments can lead to what doctors call 'clinical outcomes', or real differences in heart disease among women.

The studies which appear to demonstrate a positive outcome for HRT-users, such as the USA nurses' project, must also be viewed with caution as the 'healthy user effect' may come into play here, as in other research programmes we have mentioned. In other words, healthier lifestyles led to an interest in HRT, or doctors recommended it because the women were healthy enough to take it without problems. Dr David Ashton describes a number of these 'research' programmes as 'seriously flawed'. In some, he says, women who became unwell while taking HRT withdrew from the group, leaving only healthier women behind, in others it was found the women taking HRT had lower levels of CHD risk factors than the non-users before starting treatment. Because the rates of heart attack were likely to be much lower in these healthy subjects, it appeared the HRT was protecting them. Ashton concludes: 'It is therefore quite possible that the apparent benefits of HRT with respect to heart disease are either exaggerated or entirely absent.'

Most of the studies showing a benefit were based on women taking oestrogen alone. A small number of research programmes have shown that the combined preparation reduces the risk to the same degree, but these, like the other tests, are not conclusive and have the same flaws in their methodology. Progesterone has been said to have a positive effect on the cardiovascular system, but it could also blunt the reported positive influence of oestrogen on cholesterol.

It is obviously necessary, in order to prove whether or not HRT is useful in protecting women against heart attacks, for correctly controlled random trials to take place. A number of these are currently under way. The Million Women project mentioned earlier is due to report fully within three to five years, the WISDOM (Women's International Study of Long Duration Oestrogen After Menopause), started in 1997, will bring results in 2012, and the Women's Health Initiative (WHI), funded by the US government, also began in 1997 and will draw full conclusions in 2007.

Preliminary findings from the latter are already causing concern. In April 2000 newspapers carried headlines warning of 'Stroke risk for 1.3 million HRT women'. Only two years into the ten-year research programme, the organisers of the study involving 25,000 US women wrote to each of them, warning that they might be increasing, in small measure, their risk of strokes, heart attacks and blood clots in the lungs. Significantly they did not advise women to stop taking their HRT. Professor Maria Stefancik of the Standford Medical Centre in California who is leading part of the study said there had been 'an increase in cardio-vascular events', but emphasised that the findings were preliminary and should be treated with caution. She added that 'This highlights how little we know about a subject people think we know so much about.'

Professor Elizabeth O'Connor, head of Epidemiology at the University of California at San Diego, who is also involved in the

HRT research project, came to London in April to address a conference, and told the assembled gathering that 'While the evidence for the risk of heart attacks is not strong enough to suggest women should not take HRT, these findings certainly raise question marks over its use.' Her words were echoed by the HRT advisory service, the Amarant Trust, who issued a press release warning women 'not to panic about preliminary research into HRT/cardiac problems'. Their director, Dr Val Godfree, said there is no conclusive evidence that women taking HRT are more likely to suffer from cardiac problems and they should not come off HRT unnecessarily. She pointed out that less than 1 per cent of all volunteers on the WHI trial had experienced any problems so far and said that scientists expected the differences between women on HRT and those taking a placebo to possibly become smaller over time, as it has been established that HRT can lower cholesterol levels in women. She also pointed out that there may be difficulties with these trials in the long term as women taking part in them may be taking other forms of medication or herbal remedies which could skew the final results.

Dr Jane Somerville, emeritus professor of Cardiology at the Imperial College School of Medicine, tells me she is not overly concerned at these early findings. While she is not convinced that HRT has any role in long-term protection against heart disease, neither is she worried that it may exacerbate existing cardiac problems, except in those with a prior disposition towards thrombosis, as all oestrogens can have a role in thrombotic events. She does believe that for those women who have no known risk factors and for whom HRT relieves symptoms of tiredness, depression or severe hot flushes, the sense of wellbeing the treatment brings may be a good reason for continuing with it, especially as stress is known to be a factor in heart disease.

Nevertheless, the GP of a friend of mine in Cambridge was worried enough about the reports coming from the USA to express doubts to her patients about the wisdom of taking HRT. She demonstrates how difficult it is for responsible family doctors, who try to keep up with all the latest information about the drug, to feel confident about advising their patients on benefits and dangers until thorough long-term trials have been completed.

SIDE-EFFECTS OF HRT

Both the oestrogens and progestogens in HRT have different side-effects that you will need to bear in mind before deciding whether to take the treatment.

POSSIBLE SIDE-EFFECTS OF OESTROGENS

breast tenderness
fluid retention
nausea
nipple sensitivity
skin irritation (with patches)
vaginal discharge

These are often transient and resolve themselves without any change in treatment as time goes on. Women are encouraged to persist with each therapy for about 12 weeks to see what happens, but there is a significant short-term drop-out rate in those taking HRT. As many as two-thirds of women undertaking the treatment stop within two years, usually because of these side-effects. No matter what the long- term health or cosmetic benefits may be, there is obviously no point in taking a preparation which makes you feel crummier than you did before. It is worth sticking with the treatment and tinkering with types and doses to see if the side-effects settle down, but some women get the 'miracle cure' they hoped for, others don't and not enough is known about HRT and the individual's body chemistry to be able to make accurate predictions. If you're prepared to go through 'trial and error', go ahead, if not, don't feel bad about quitting.

Nausea with oral HRT can be helped by adjusting the timing of the dose or taking it with food. (Edwina Currie takes hers in the morning and then goes back to bed for half an hour to let things settle down.) Nausea may also be due to a lactose sensitivity, in which case a different form of HRT may be necessary. Synthetic oestrogens or conjugated equine oestrogens may cause more sickness.

Breast tenderness may be relieved by taking a supplement of oil of evening primrose. Dr Hilary Jones suggests reducing salt intake and cutting out tea and coffee.

POSSIBLE SIDE-EFFECTS OF PROGESTOGENS

The side-effects of progestogens can be both physical and psychological.

Physical effects	Psychological effects
abdominal cramps	aggression
acne	anxiety
backache	apathy
breast tenderness	confusion
clumsiness	depression
dizziness	difficulty making decisions
fluid retention	feeling irrational
general aches and pains	forgetfulness
greasy skin	irritability
headaches	panic attacks
poor sleep	poor concentration
tiredness	restlessness
weight gain	tearfulness

These side-effects are believed to be connected to the type, duration and dose of progestogen – you'll remember that Edwina found her dose was too high initially and the progestogen gave her spots and increased aggression. Strategies doctors may recommend are:

- changing the type from a C19 (testosterone-based) to a C21 (progesterone-based) progestogen
- trying a vaginal method, a patch or a Mirena
- reducing duration, but within the 10–14 days a month required for endometrial protection
- using the three-monthly bleed HRT or the continuous combined (no-bleed) HRT which are only suitable for post-menopausal women.

Irregular breakthough bleeding should be investigated, but it can occur in the following cases:

- if HRT is not taken as prescribed or if its effect has been reduced by other medication or as a result of a stomach upset
- if the long cycle (bleed every three months) type is taken, breakthrough bleeding can occur in the first couple of months
- in continuous combined HRT, light bleeding or spotting is common in the first three to six months of treatment, but if pelvic discomfort or heavy bleeding occurs, further investigation is necessary.

As the bleeding is related to progestogen, doctors may again wish to change the dose or the type taken.

WEIGHT GAIN

Virtually every woman I've spoken to who is otherwise satisfied with her HRT will say it caused her to put on weight. My anecdotal evidence is borne out by Marilyn Glenville, who is an expert on alternatives to HRT. Many of the women she sees say they have put on weight because of the drug. Even Teresa Gorman, the most ardent exponent of the therapy, says her weight went up considerably and she has a photo of herself in which, she says, she looks like a leg of pork. She dieted seriously to get back to something closer to her old weight, but says she wouldn't want to be too skinny. It may be glamorous to be stick-thin (it was Wallis Simpson who had embroidered on one of her cushions 'You can never be too rich or too thin'), but it's very ageing. Edwina Currie battles constantly with an extra half-stone and Joan Bakewell has a similar problem. I, as you know, am with Teresa on this one as I think a little extra covering can help to fill out wrinkles beautifully.

There is no clinical evidence that the weight gain is caused by the HRT and there is no doubt that post-menopausal women tend to gain weight anyway as the metabolism slows, so less food is needed to keep going. Also, the body's fat distribution tends to go through a natural change so that weight is gained around the waist and abdomen and lost on the hips and thighs.

A small research programme, involving 560 women, carried out at St Thomas' Hospital in London in 1996, found those taking HRT had less body fat overall than those not taking HRT and had 9 per cent less fat around the abdomen. Katherine Samaras, the Australian endocrinologist who carried out the research, said this reported change in fat distribution may have an influence on heart disease, but it is not clear whether or not there was a healthy-user effect in this test. It could be the case that the HRT-users were more appearance-conscious and watched their weight more carefully than those who were not taking the treatment.

RISKS OF HRT

There are several potential risks associated with HRT. Make sure you discuss these with your doctor before starting treatment.

VENOUS THROMBO-EMBOLISM

Until recently HRT, unlike the contraceptive pill, was not thought to increase the risk of blood clots, which in up to 2 per cent of cases can be fatal, but a series of recent studies shows the risk is slightly increased.

Out of 10,000 women not taking HRT, one would be expected to develop a thrombosis. This risk increases to three in 10,000 for women on HRT. To balance the level of danger, for women in normal pregnancy the risk is six out of every 10,000 women. One study has suggested the risk is restricted to the first year of HRT use, raising the possibility that HRT reacts with a previously undiagnosed risk of thrombosis.

These studies underline the importance of telling your doctor everything you can about your medical history and lifestyle in order for a proper assessment to be made before a decision is taken on whether HRT would suit you or not. A strong family history, previous thrombosis or severe varicose veins would obviously be good reasons for not embarking on HRT.

BREAST CANCER

Most of the body's cells are replaced lots of times during a lifetime. The new cells are exact replicas and are produced only when needed, but problems can arise if they become genetically altered during division. Errors can be picked up by the body's own system and corrected, but occasionally they are not detected, and those cells which are not checked by the normal mechanisms can grow into cancer.

As the body grows older it becomes less efficient at correcting mistakes, but other factors can cause damage to the DNA and make cancer more likely. Smoking is the best known environmental element that has this effect.

It is not known how breast cancer is caused, but it is probably a combination of things. One of these is hormonal stimulation. It is known that women who begin their periods at an early age (before 12) and finish them later in life (after 55) have a increased risk of developing the disease. Also in a higher risk group are women who have never had children or start to have them over the age of 30.

This is thought to be because the woman's breast is exposed to oestrogen for longer. Oestrogen encourages the cells in the breast to multiply, and the more oestrogen that's floating around, the more often and more speedily the cells replicate themselves. If the speed and frequency of multiplication is too high, there is more room for error. The more damaged cells there are, the more difficult it becomes for the body's own immune system to deal with them efficiently. If the mutated cells divide before they are eliminated by the immune system then breast cancer can develop. Thus oestrogen is not a direct cause of the cancer, but it does create the environment in which cancer can develop.

This knowledge led logically to the theory that HRT, which adds oestrogen to the body beyond its normal life cycle, could cause breast cancer. Conflicting research existed for a number of years until, in 1997, a huge analysis was published which gave the results of a re-assessment of 90 per cent of all the worldwide data on HRT and breast cancer risk. It was carried out by Professor Valerie Beral of the Imperial Cancer Research Fund Epidemiology

Unit in Oxford, who is also responsible for co-ordinating the British Million Women Study.

Beral's initial research showed that for women aged 50 not using HRT around 45 in every 1000 will have breast cancer diagnosed over the next 20 years.

The additional risks for women using HRT are:
- 5 years' use: the figure rises by 2 to 47 in every 1000
- 10 years' use: rises by 6 to 51 in every 1000
- 15 years' use: rises by 12 to 57 in every 1000

If HRT is taken for more than five years, the individual risk of each woman must be weighed against the benefits of continuing on HRT. Those with a high risk of osteoporosis, in the light of current evidence about the need to take the treatment long term for any real benefit to accrue at the period of highest risk in the sixties and seventies, will need to make a careful balance of risk versus benefit.

Teresa Gorman is clear about her decision to take HRT, probably for the rest of her life. While she is not in a high-risk group for osteoporosis, she believes she has seen enormous benefits from taking HRT. She cites her energy levels, lack of aches and pains, good skin and hair quality as vital components in her ability to continue with her job as an MP throughout her fifties and sixties. Now at 67 she feels as well as she did in her forties. If, she told me, she were diagnosed with breast cancer tomorrow, she would still be grateful for the 17 years of extreme wellbeing she attributes to the treatment. For her, it was a risk worth taking.

In addition, research has shown that women who develop breast cancer while on HRT appear more likely to survive the disease. Initial studies found a 16 per cent reduction in mortality in HRT-users and the first results from the Million Women Study, published in October 2000, are encouraging. The study was set up in 1996 and recruited women from routine breast cancer screening when they were called through the National Health Screening Programme. Britain is the only country in the world which can carry out such a study, because of its unique combination of a large population and comprehensive breast-screening programme.

The primary aim of the research is to establish the effects of use of different types of HRT on the risk of developing breast cancer. More than a million volunteers offered to take part, which is one in four of all women in the UK aged 50 to 65. The early results show that of all women in that age group in the UK, half have used HRT at some time and one in 70 has had breast cancer and survived. One of the researchers said of these findings, 'About 70,000 women aged 50 to 65 in the UK are living with breast cancer; although large numbers of women have had the disease, many are surviving for long periods of time.'

Breast screening on HRT
HRT use is not seen as a special case for breast screening. All women aged 50 to 65 are being invited every two years, although as I mentioned earlier there is debate about whether this should be extended to older women and the head of the screening service has said no woman of whatever age would be turned away if she requested a mammogram. There is evidence that breast cancer is harder to detect in women who take HRT. After the menopause, breast tissue naturally becomes less dense and any tumour is relatively easy to detect. On HRT the tissue is cloudier and mammograms are more difficult to interpret, as they would be in a younger woman. Women on HRT may therefore be prone to more false positives and be recalled after screening.

There is some controversy as to whether women should always have a mammogram before taking HRT, to allow radiographers to make later comparisions. In the USA, HRT is only given after a normal mammogram, although this practice is not routine in Britain. Dr Marion Everitt in the Leeds Menopause Clinic is a supporter of a health MOT before prescribing HRT and is supported by a number of other doctors in the field. If you want one, ask.

Younger women and breast cancer with hormone treatment
Younger women who lack hormones after a natural early menopause (before 40) or who lost them because of the need to have a hysterectomy when young, have a low risk of breast cancer, as a result, it's thought, of their low exposure to their own oestrogen. Doctors believe that HRT merely returns them to a risk level which is roughly equivalent to what it would have been under normal circumstances. These women will only begin to have an extra risk of breast cancer after the age of 50, and then only in the same way as other women on HRT after the menopause.

This has not been the subject of extra research, as it's difficult to find large numbers of women in this position and to follow them over a period of time, so it's just an educated guess, but doctors are convinced that women in this position do need hormones because they have a greater risk of osteoporosis than women who experience a normal menopause.

Gail Jones, who had her menopause in her mid-twenties, has no doubts about taking HRT. What turned out to be normal menopausal symptoms, she had thought were signs of a life-threatening disease. When her early menopause was diagnosed, she was relieved that she was not going to die. She, more than anyone, is convinced that her feelings of depression, hot flushes, dry skin, tiredness and heavy bleeding were not 'all in the mind'. How could they be? she says, when the last thing she was expecting was the menopause, even though the symptoms were classic.

Gail describes her HRT as giving her back her life. It made her start feeling like a young person again and she has no qualms about taking it for ever. Whatever risks there are, she feels, are more than outweighed by the benefits. She has a breast check every six months and is aware that the risk of breast cancer increases with age and HRT use, but she is balanced in her view of it. 'So what if they do find breast cancer?' she told me. 'It might have been there anyway. This way, the plea I made to God when I thought I was dying, to let me live to 40 to look after my kids, has been more than fulfilled.'

The progestogen question

There is a problem with the analysis above in that the majority of research thus far has been carried out on women on oestrogen-only HRT. The effects of combined HRT may increase the risk of breast cancer even further.

Two studies carried out in the United States and published early in 2000 both found evidence of increased incidence of breast cancer in women who were taking both oestrogen and progestogen. The most recent research, conducted at the University of Southern California found a 24 per cent increase in risk for every five years of use. Researchers found a higher breast cancer risk in women who only took progestogen for part of the month and concluded that continuous combined HRT may be better overall as the doses of progestogen tend to be lower. This again is an area about which there can't be said to be conclusive knowledge until the results of longer term work are known.

With regard to breast cancer, the Million Women Study will ask:

- What effects do combined oestrogen and progestogen therapy have on breast cancer risk?
- Are breast cancers detected at screening in women who have used HRT or oral contraceptives different in terms of size and invasiveness than the cancers detected in women who have never used these hormones?

- How does HRT use affect the efficacy of breast cancer screening?
- How does HRT use affect mortality from breast cancer and other conditions?

More useful data should be available in three years' time.

REPRODUCTIVE CANCERS

It is well proven that the addition of an adequate dose of progestogen for women who have not had a hysterectomy reduces the risk of endometrial cancer to the same level as for those who do not use HRT. Some studies have suggested it reduces the risk even further.

There is no significant evidence to show that HRT increases the risks of ovarian or cervical cancer, which are more common than endometrial cancer, nor that HRT should be withheld if women have these cancers. Again, more research is needed as some studies found a weak link between HRT and ovarian cancer, while others found no link at all. There is some evidence that HRT reduces the incidence of colonic cancers.

THE PROBLEM WITH MEDICAL STUDIES

Most doctors will argue – indeed, it is increasingly a requirement within the NHS – that they can only practise 'evidence-based medicine', but, as we've seen already, there are lots of difficulties in assessing the quality of research and balancing frankly conflicting reports, whether the medication under consideration is conventional HRT or the many alternatives which will be discussed in the next chapter.

We have already seen the problems caused when the 'healthy-user effect' is not taken into account by researchers. Equally, the most respected form of trial – the prospective random controlled trial – can present difficulties. In this case participants are chosen at random – by computer, rather than, say, in the USA nurses' study, where they were selected from one sector of society where people may take more care of their health than in others. There are ethical questions in relation to randomisation. Is it fair, for instance, if a study is to be carried out over a long period, to deny one group a treatment which may do them good?

Monitoring prospectively, rather than retrospectively, means following people into the future. It is believed to be more reliable than asking them to remember the past, as memory can play tricks and we tend to remember the bad more graphically than the good.

A controlled trial compares a group that receives treatment with a control group that doesn't. If the trial is double blind, neither the participants nor the researchers know who is taking the real treatment and who is taking a placebo (a fake treatment). This is important to ensure that the researchers do not make assumptions on the basis of class, creed, or state of health of the subject, but it can still be unreliable. The placebo effect is very common in relation to hot flushes with a lot of women reporting relief with dummy pills. In some trials the effect was shown to be almost as great as HRT. If this is the result of women becoming more relaxed because they think they are taking something that will help, it may be an argument for relaxation classes.

A number of the studies carried out are described as 'under-powered'. In other words, not enough people were studied to make a significant statistical result. It was because of this that Professor Valerie Beral put together a number of studies carried out across the world in order to arrive at more reliable statistics on breast cancer risk.

These limitations on the quality of medical research lead doctors to a position where they have to make decisions on the precautionary principle. Some believe that the horrors of diseases such as osteoporosis are significant enough for large numbers of women to suggest HRT should be prescribed for the majority, even though there may be some risk of thrombosis or breast cancer for the few. Some people disagree with this approach, saying that women are being pressed into taking drugs which may keep them mobile in order to save themselves from becoming a burden on the state. Others have argued that the risks of HRT have been swept under the carpet simply because of commercial pressures. These debates will no doubt continue among doctors' organisations, information services and women-led self-help groups.

In *The Menopause, HRT and You* Caroline Hawkridge points to a worrying possibility for the future:

> *These arguments suggest it could be a short step to blaming women who do not comply with HRT. What is known as the 'Victim blaming attitude' is already well established towards smokers, unhealthy eaters and others who appear to be negligent about lifestyle advice, in spite of the powerful commercial lobbies and social pressures that encourage their behaviour.*

There is evidence that this is happening already. The novelist Maggie Grahame told me about a friend of hers who had two heart attacks in her early fifties and was rebuked by the cardiologists who took care of her for not having taken HRT, despite the fact that she had already told them that her diet was 'lousy', she smoked 40 cigarettes a day, was prevented from doing exercise by a crippling spine condition and the possible benefits of HRT in relation to heart disease are strongly disputed.

NEGATIVE EXPERIENCES OF HRT

Just as we must be cautious about the reports of medical studies which proclaim either the benefits or negative effects of HRT, so too we should weigh up carefully some of the anecdotal opposition or over-enthusiasm that is frequently bandied about.

- **Women whose HRT doesn't suit them**
  It is a fact that 25 per cent of women who take HRT stop within the first six months. Some, like Eve Pollard, may be women who have had experience of oestrogen before, decide it's not for them and are content with their decision. Others need to find sympathetic and well informed practitioners who will jiggle treatments to find a suitable one.
- **Women who expect too much**
  A common theme that emerges is the need to dispel the idea that HRT is the elixir of youth, because inevitably a lot of women will be disappointed.
- **Women who are made ill by HRT**
  It is acknowledged that a certain proportion of women with HRT will not tolerate it because the known side effects such as painful breasts, PMS, bloating, etc are too unpleasant.

There are some women who claim HRT has given them unusual and distressing illnesses which doctors cannot agree are caused by HRT. There is one group – Doctors Against the Abuse of Sex Steroid Hormones (DASH) – that has consistently opposed the treatment and voices its concerns regularly to the *British Medical Journal* about the safety of HRT, rightly calling for women to be properly informed about the risks. The honorary secretary of DASH, Ellen Grant, is a consultant in nutrition, migraines and allergies and believes the risks of HRT are greater than is generally estimated, but feels they do not emerge because research money is often directed at the wrong people. In her opinion, the menopause can be aided by helping to re-balance the body naturally, through nutrition (more about this in Chapter 7).

One of the loudest exponents of this view of HRT as a danger to women's health is Maggie Tuttle, who runs her own Menopausal Helpline and claims 10,000 women have called her since 1995 with a variety of symptoms from hair loss to suicidal tendencies. When I spoke to Maggie, she told me she had been given HRT in her mid-thirties after suffering depression when she lost a baby, so she is untypical in that her symptoms cannot be said to have been those of the peri- or post-menopausal woman. She says she took the treatment for 15 years and had problems with headaches, thinning hair, memory, rashes, a burning sensation, pains in the neck and shoulders and red eyes. She also says bone density tests revealed thinning in her bones.

Maggie's helpline asks women who phone in to send a £5 cheque, in exchange for which they will receive an information pack. The information included in the pack is resolutely anti-HRT and pro certain alternative therapies. The helpline offers an ordering service for items such as dong quai, coral calcium, Linda Kearns' cake, St John's wort, red clover, lecithin and various vitamins. Natural progesterone cream (see p. 183) is also suggested. The only medically recognised and reportedly effective form of this treatment is licensed in Britain exclusively on prescription, as it is a hormone. The name of Dr Paul Layman is mentioned in the helpline's literature in relation to natural progesterone. I spoke to him and he tells me an increasing number of conventionally trained doctors are now willing to prescribe the cream. He explained that he conducts consultations over the phone and pointed out that it is possible to obtain the product by mail order from other countries where it is not regulated, such as South Africa, the USA or the Irish Republic. It is up to you to decide whether or not this form of self-medication can to be adequately monitored. All these alternative treatments are discussed more fully in Chapter 6.

There are women who have suffered from the known risks of HRT such as breast cancer or blood clots. In April 2000 Pat Mitchell's compensation of £40,000 was reported in the newspapers. She won her claim after alleging that she had been put on HRT without her knowledge and subsequently contracted breast cancer. She said she had been given an implant in hospital in 1973 after an operation which resulted in her having her womb and one ovary removed.

In 1998 the first death in which HRT was cited as the cause was reported. Irene Brankin was given the treatment in her mid-forties and died within three months of starting it. Her husband, Bernard, alleges that she suffered dizzy spells within weeks, but was advised to continue. Nine weeks after beginning the treatment she had a seizure and died later in hospital after surgery to remove a blood clot on her lung. The coroner concluded that HRT was the cause of death.

When incidents like these occur it can be for a number of reasons.

- Women who suffer in this way may have balanced benefit and risk and become one of the statistics we know about. They were fully informed of the potential problems and may or may not have had a condition which would predispose them to cancer or cardiac trouble. Just like driving a car, we know the risks, but take them anyway.
- Some women may have been more at risk because they were unsuitable for HRT in the first place and either their medical history was not properly assessed or they were economical with the truth during assessment.
- HRT may have been administered negligently; for example, a woman may have been given too many implants without blood levels being checked.

So what should I do?

It will be a few years yet before we really know the benefits or otherwise of taking Hormone Replacement Therapy. Until then, we're all just guinea pigs in what may prove to be the greatest or the worst thing for women's health in our middle, post-reproductive years.

It is obviously not good enough for doctors to dish out packages of pills which are not designed for your complex individual body chemistry. It's cavalier of them to toss out glibly, 'What do you want, pills or patches?' or, at the other extreme, to ask, 'What do you want it for, our grandmothers managed without it?' A doctor's job is to treat you as an individual with thoughts, knowledge, feelings and values as well as blood, bone, heart and hormones.

Armed with the information in Chapters 4 and 5, think carefully before going to your GP about the kind of older woman you want to be. (We'll discuss this in detail in the final chapter.) Are your skin, hair and the energy to keep up with a fast-moving world important to you or are you ready for a more relaxed approach to life? Do you want to look youthful or would you prefer to grow into your wrinkles and greying hair? Are you convinced by the osteoporosis evidence? How do you feel about the heart disease research? Will you worry every time you take a tablet about breast cancer or are you more like Teresa Gorman, prepared to be pragmatic about the slightly increased risk in favour of other benefits?

Think, too, about the kind of woman you have been. What is your medical history and that of your family? Dr Val Godfree of the Amarant Trust told me that some women are less than honest about contra-indications because they are so keen to get HRT. One woman who developed blinding headaches on the treatment had failed to inform her doctor of a previous history of migraines. Do you exercise? Do you smoke or drink? When you had your babies were you keen to have every pain-killer and monitor known to modern science or did you want a more natural form of childbirth? Did you take the pill as a contraceptive without a second thought or were you happier to put up with less convenient methods of contraception because you hated the thought of taking drugs that would alter your body's chemistry for a long period?

Glenda Jackson told me she'd have a nervous breakdown if she took so much as an aspirin – all she has in her medicine cupboard is TCP and plasters. Linda Taylor, the pop singer, hates tablets so much she doesn't even take antibiotics. Angela Mason, from the Stonewall organisation, on the other hand, says she has no relationship whatsoever with her body. She simply wants it to function enough to enable her to get on with her job and look after her teenage daughter. When her doctor offered her pills she took them, they worked and she asked no questions at all. The radio and TV presenter Gloria Hunniford has taken vitamins all her life, but feels uneasy about taking drugs. She prefers to wait until she really needs them, say to keep a life-threatening condition under control.

The only thing that counts in all this is how *you* feel. Doctors don't know how you feel, you do and you shouldn't be bamboozled either way by practitioners who are propagandists for the therapy or those who think the whole HRT business is a waste of NHS resources to serve a bunch of neurotic middle-aged women. Both extremes are wrong and whether you take HRT or not is your choice, not theirs. And your views may change. If symptoms become too much to bear you can, as have some of the women we've discussed, take a treatment for a short while and then pack it in. You can chop and change until you find something that suits or you can decide to take nothing now and revise your opinion at a later date.

What some doctors won't do is prescribe alternative or complementary medicines. Doctors in the NHS have to practise evidence-based medicine and, as we've seen, it's tough enough for them to do that on the basis of conflicting and inconclusive studies currently available on HRT. Dr Marion Everitt in Leeds refuses to deal with alternatives because, she says, there is no convincing data to show any of them works, they are expensive to buy and she worries that over-the-counter remedies may be dangerous, as we've seen in some cases with Chinese herbal medicines. She says they are not tried, tested or quality controlled to the same level as pharmaceuticals.

So, are alternatives any safer or more efficacious than conventional HRT and if you chose to take them, under whose care should you do it? . . .

CHAPTER 6

THE ALTERNATIVES TO HRT

HRT has had plenty of glowingly healthy and youthful looking exponents, Joan Bakewell and Teresa Gorman among them, but complementary therapies have their role models too. Gloria Hunniford, the TV and radio presenter, is 60 now and couldn't look better. She has the energy to work 17-hour days three times a week and swears by her regime of homeopathic medicines, vitamins (pure E for the arteries and skin, 1000 mg C for all-round wellbeing), evening primrose oil, Osteoprime and Urtcalcium (for bones – she suffered a serious fracture in her shoulder when she was 50), Celatron Tri Plus 3 (Barbara Cartland's favourite 'brain pill') and a product called Female Balance.

Gloria says she didn't rule out HRT, but was one of those fortunate women who had no symptoms, her periods just stopped. She still holds it in reserve should she need it in the future for bone density, but she developed her attitudes and medication with the help of Jan de Vries, a homeopath, osteopath and naturopath she met at Radio 2 in 1982. Before that she had taken only one multivitamin. Sensibly, she does not self-medicate, but works under the guidance of a qualified practitioner.

British women are less likely to use HRT than our European

counterparts (25 per cent of us currently, as opposed to 55 per cent of French women and an even higher European average) but we are most likely to take the so-called natural therapies. Surveys suggest 16 per cent of women in Britain take them compared with a European average of 10 per cent.

Natural therapies can range from those simulating natural hormones to complementary practices such as herbalism, acupuncture and homoeopathy.

NATURAL PROGESTERONE

This is the most talked about of all the complementary therapies and its best-known promoter is a Californian doctor, John Lee, the author of *What Your Doctor May Not Tell You About Menopause*.

Lee challenges head-on the received wisdom that troublesome menopausal symptoms are the result of oestrogen deficiency and says, on the contrary, that it is a lack of progesterone that causes hot flushes, night sweats and all the other attendant miseries at the time of the menopause, together with longer-term health problems.

He argues that at the menopause the oestrogen level declines, but we carry on producing it in smaller amounts from the adrenal glands and in the body fat and muscle cells. Those of us who are plumper will carry on producing our own oestrogen longer than our thinner counterparts, but the average oestrogen drop is by one-half or a third. Progesterone levels, on the other hand, sink close to zero because we no longer ovulate, so the production of progesterone by the corpus luteum ceases to be triggered. Levels of progesterone are, on average, $\frac{1}{120}$th of what they were.

Throughout a woman's fertile life, progesterone has balanced oestrogen – most apparently, as we've discussed, in the preparation of the lining of the womb for ovulation and pregnancy. Dr Lee lists a number of other ways, quoted in *Natural Progesterone*, Dr Shirley Bond and Anna Rushton's book on natural progesterone, in which the two hormones work together.

The effects of oestrogen
  aids salt and fluid retention
  breast stimulation
  causes endometrial cancer
  contributes to depression and headaches
  contributes to the loss of zinc and retention of copper
  decreases libido
  impairs blood sugar control
  increases blood clotting
  increases body fat
  increases risk of breast cancer
  interferes with thyroid hormone
  reduces oxygen levels in all cells
  reduces vascular tone
  slightly restrains osteoclast function in order to slow down bone loss
  triggers auto-immune disease

The effects of progesterone
  helps prevent breast cancer
  helps use fat for energy
  improves vascular tone
  increases libido
  facilitates thyroid hormone action
  natural anti-depressant
  natural diuretic
  necessary for survival of embryo
  normalises blood clotting
  normalises blood sugar levels
  normalises zinc and copper levels

precursor of corticosterone production
prevents endometrial cancer
protects against fibrocystic breasts
restores proper cell oxygen levels
stimulates osteoblast bone building
turns off auto-immune diseases

OESTROGEN DOMINANCE

John Lee believes that at the time of the menopause many women are suffering not from oestrogen deficiency, but oestrogen dominance, and that it is when the two hormones are unbalanced that problems occur. Oestrogen, he says, can be high or low, but the dominance refers to its level relative to progesterone.

The theory says that the main culprits responsible for oestrogen dominance are xeno-oestrogens which exist in the environment and come from pesticides, herbicides, insecticides and the breakdown products of processes in the petrochemicals and plastics industries. They are believed to seep from plastics, paints and chemicals in some cosmetics and are thought to be stored in animal fat. These chemicals have the characteristic of behaving like oestrogens and can attach themselves to the oestrogen receptors in the body. They are said to have potent effects and to be difficult for the body to remove.

We know from Chapter 1 that during the perimenopause irregular and heavy periods can be caused because we have ceased to ovulate and the ovaries produce oestrogen, but no progesterone because no egg is released. When the lining of the womb is stimulated by oestrogen alone and without monthly periodic shedding brought about by progesterone, the tissue continues to proliferate until it outgrows its blood supply, causing the irregular bleed. Lee's theory is that xeno-oestrogens can bring about this problem even before the perimenopause, causing women to use up the eggs in their ovaries too quickly and reach a state of burn-out in their late thirties or early forties, whereby they produce oestrogen, but no progesterone for a longer time than would be expected. This effect can be exacerbated by stress or poor diet. So oestrogen dominance can occur as a combination of factors, some of which are entirely the result of modern living: extra hormones from the environment and an inadequate diet which cannot buffer the changes. So it's not the fault of nature, but our own.

Symptoms of oestrogen dominance (according to Dr John Lee)
   acceleration of the ageing process
   allergies, including asthma, rashes, sinus congestion
   auto-immune disorders
   breast tenderness
   cervical dysplasia
   cold hands and feet, relating to thyroid dysfunction
   decreased sex drive
   depression with anxiety or agitation
   dry eyes
   early onset of menstruation
   fat gain, especially about the abdomen, hips and thighs
   fatigue
   fibrocystic breasts
   gall bladder disease
   hair loss
   headaches
   hypoglycaemia
   inability to focus
   increased blood clotting
   increased risk of strokes
   infertility
   insomnia
   irregular menstruation

irritability
memory loss
miscarriage
mood swings
osteoporosis
PMS
pre-menopausal bone loss
sluggish metabolism
uterine cancer
uterine fibroids
water retention, bloating

At the menopause, night sweats, hot flushes, dry vagina and mood swings are seen as a direct result of the imbalance between oestrogen and progesterone.

Dr Adam Carey, who is a gynaecologist at the Reproductive Medicine Trust, is currently running trials on natural progesterone's possible role in controlling hot flushes and bone-thinning. Carey finds the idea of oestrogen dominance an interesting concept. He says it's an oversimplification to say it would throw everything out of balance, and is not convinced by the long list of symptoms put forward by Lee, but says the idea that we need some balance between the two hormones is not as wild as it sounds.

As far as xeno-oestrogens are concerned, he agrees that such chemicals in the environment will have an effect on the body, not because they are oestrogens in themselves, but because they may, for example, affect the liver and the way it breaks down oestrogen.

He believes that historically people have overlooked progesterone. It was only added to conventional HRT when the endometrial cancer problem raised its head. After all the work done on perfecting a progestogen that could be absorbed orally it was unlikely, he says, that the pharmaceutical companies would then make a further investment in a natural alternative. He suggests that progestogens have modified natural molecules which can be patented. The ingredient in natural progesterone cannot be patented and is open to anyone to develop.

WHAT IS 'NATURAL' PROGESTERONE?

As we know from earlier chapters, most HRT uses progestogens rather than natural progesterone because the latter is difficult to take orally and doesn't dissolve well in patches. There are some natural progesterone products available on the market and classed as conventional HRT – Crinone (see p. 127) is one I mentioned earlier – but it's argued that the dose provided in these cases is 10 to 20 times higher than the ovaries would naturally supply. Dr Lee's research is based on prescribing progesterone at the normal physiological level, albeit based on pre-menopausal amounts.

Natural progesterone is most commonly made from a substance called diosgenin, which is found most prolifically in wild yams, extracted and synthesised in the laboratory. We're back to that word 'natural' again, which means nothing more in this case, as in the case of 'natural' oestrogens and progesterone in HRT, than that scientists have managed to manufacture a hormonal substance which has the same chemical structure as that in the body. Progesterone is NOT present in the wild yam or in soy, but diosgenin is. The body does not have the enzymes to convert the substance into progesterone from the food product. So you have to be careful. When we first mentioned 'natural' progesterone on *Woman's Hour* a couple of years ago, I was inundated with little pots of wild yam cream from a number of companies making 'wild' claims for its properties in helping the menopausal woman. Basically, if you can buy it over the counter or by mail order legitimately in this country it's unlikely to be the real stuff. Progest is the familiar brand name for natural progesterone in this country and must, as I have already pointed out, be obtained on prescription and supervised by a doctor.

Headlines which warn against the 'wild yam scam' may be a little exaggerated as the plant itself is said to have a number of properties. It is anti-spasmodic, sedative, anti-inflammatory and it can nourish the adrenal glands which can then make small amounts of progesterone, although not from the wild yam itself.

How natural progesterone is used

Unlike other hormonal preparations, natural progesterone doesn't dissolve in alcohol, but can be dissolved in vitamin E and is generally applied as skin cream. The recommendation is that you should rub it into any part of the skin – apart from on the breasts – and rotate the sites daily. It is believed to be absorbed well through the skin into the fat cells and the bloodstream (although the King's College Research disputes this, see opposite).

Dr Lee believes a good progesterone cream should provide about 400–500mg of natural progesterone per ounce which will supply around 20–30mg of dosage per day. Pre-menopausal women naturally produce 5–10mg per day prior to ovulation and 20–50mg after ovulation. In pregnant women, levels can reach upto 400mg per day. Be careful, as mentioned above, to get the right sort of cream. This should only apply if you are not going through a doctor, but using mail order or other countries as your source. Some of what Dr Shirley Bond describes as 'home-made creams' do not have the micronised form of progesterone in them and so won't be effective. The amount of natural progesterone varies so you need to check the label. Some creams may also contain other substances, including oestrogen or phyto-oestrogen, but you won't want this if you're trying to combat oestrogen dominance.

Dr Lee is not against women using oestrogen if symptoms such as hot flushes are not controlled by the progesterone alone, although the use of progesterone with conventional HRT is not recommended by the Amarant Trust, following the King's College Research (see opposite).

Dr Bond says it is very difficult to overdose using the cream, although it may be possible to have too much of the oral or vaginal forms. It can be used as soon as symptoms begin during the perimenopause and for as long as you wish. She says there are no reported side effects with natural progesterone cream, although in the early days of use women may experience breast tenderness, headaches or depression. This is rare and generally passes after the first month. There are some women who will find it doesn't suit them, as with any hormone treatment. If you don't feel right on it, stop.

NATURAL PROGESTERONE WHERE HRT IS UNSUITABLE

Some doctors are willing to prescribe natural progesterone as an alternative for women who either cannot tolerate HRT or for whom it is not advisable. I have only come across doctors in the private sector – notably, Dr Shirley Bond (the author, with Anna Rushton, of a book on the subject) in Harley Street. I am told some GPs will prescribe it if you can persuade them or if they and the health authority are convinced of its efficacy. You will generally have to pay for the prescription privately and for supplies as there is little evidence of natural progesterone being available on the NHS. As it is a hormone, it is unwise to use it without the supervision of a qualified doctor.

It is vital that women who have not had a hysterectomy but are taking oestrogen HRT, should not attempt to use natural progesterone in place of the prescribed progestogen used to oppose their oestrogen. In 1997, the King's College Hospital Trust, together with a number of other menopause clinics and the

Amarant Trust, discovered that some women were doing this, having ordered their natural progesterone from the USA or Ireland, and were having problems with the endometrium. Both trusts commissioned a trial using Progest to assess absorption, metabolism and urinary excretion and found the body's absorption of the hormone was relatively low. They concluded that Progest should not be substituted for conventional progestogen as it will not protect the endometrium from stimulation by oestrogen. They also said that it would have no effect in protection against osteoporosis (see p. 188), although some people have argued that their results cannot be relied upon. They tested only 20 women over a 30-day period and checked the body's uptake of the hormone through blood tests, which supporters of natural progesterone say is not as accurate as a saliva test. Nevertheless, mixing and matching your own treatments is not to be recommended.

Advocates of natural progesterone claim that it can help in the following conditions.

Fibroids and endometriosis
Natural progesterone can be useful for women with fibroids, which can be seen as a problem of oestrogen dominance. Taking HRT can be a problem for women with fibroids as oestrogen can stimulate their growth. Natural progesterone is said not to reduce fibroids, but may stop them from getting larger.

Endometriosis can also start up again in a small number of cases when women take HRT. Natural progesterone does not carry this risk and may, therefore, be an alternative. Some women have reported an improvement in their condition whilst taking natural progesterone, but the evidence is anecdotal.

The synthetic progestogens used to oppose oestrogen in conventional HRT are not thought to be useful in cases of fibroids or endometriosis, even though they can successfully protect against endometrial cancer. It's argued that synthetic progestogens are not capable of matching the full range of progesterone's functions. They may even reduce the efficacy of what remains of the body's own progesterone because, by attaching to the receptor sites, they may block the ability of the natural hormone to carry out its functions.

Hot flushes

An American study published in the *Journal of Obstetrics and Gynaecology* in 1999 suggested that natural progesterone cream may reduce or completely relieve hot flushes. In the double-blind, placebo-controlled study, 83 per cent of the women who applied 20mg of progesterone in cream form each day had either an improvement or complete resolution of hot flushes. More studies are underway.

Breast cancer

We have already seen that the progestogen component of conventional HRT may increase the risk of breast cancer, although the results of trials are awaited. Dr Shirley Bond argues that natural progesterone may protect against breast cancer as it reduces proliferation of the breast tissue. She goes on to say:

> Work has been published that shows that women being operated on for breast cancer who have high levels of progesterone both at the time of the surgery and afterwards show dramatically improved survival rates. From this point of view, wherever possible, women should try to schedule any surgery in the second half of their menstrual cycle when progesterone levels are high. The 30-year retrospective study done at Johns Hopkins University in the US found that women who were low in progesterone had 5.4 times more incidence of breast cancer and 10 times more deaths from cancer of all kinds. Also, a French study, published in the Journal

of Fertility and Sterility *showed that the value of progesterone lies in the fact that it actually slows down the rate at which cell division occurs in the breast ducts.*

There is as yet no evidence from controlled double-blind prospective medical trials to show whether the claims that natural progesterone can protect against breast cancer or aid in recovery can be made with confidence, although Suzannah Olivier, author of *The Breast Cancer Prevention and Recovery Diet*, refers to animal studies which confirm it may be useful in combating oestrogen dominance. She says that Dr John Lee has been using it for 20 years in the management of breast cancer.

Professor Valerie Beral of the Million Women Study is dismissive of the treatment. She says there is no adequate data on natural progesterone to know whether it would influence breast cancer one way or another. In the Million Women Study, fewer than 1000 women are taking natural progesterone and Professor Beral says its use is based on the spreading of rumours and folklore and that we are long way from large-scale investigation. Its supporters would argue that this lack of academically acceptable data is caused by lack of investment in trials, because the big money comes from the pharmaceutical industry which has had no interest in it.

Osteoporosis

The theory is that, while oestrogen slows down bone loss, it is progesterone that stimulates the osteoblasts that build new bone. Advocates of natural progesterone believe it can guard against osteoporosis and help to build bone density along with other dietary and exercise improvements.

Dr Lee discovered that while treating menopausal women who had been unable to take oestrogen with natural progesterone, bone scans showed that bone density increased. In his own trials which have been published in medical journals he says his patients showed a 10 per cent increase in the first year, followed by 3 to 5 per cent each following year.

The King's College trial was a double-blind placebo-controlled test, which I mentioned earlier in relation to the protection of the lining of the womb. The research team found very low levels of progesterone in the bloodstream of Progest-takers, even though the women took two to four times the recommended dose. They commented that a 2oz jar of cream contained only 200mg of progesterone and said absorption levels were probably too low to have any biological effect and could not save bone density. As I said earlier, supporters have disputed the findings, arguing that saliva tests would have been more sensitive than blood tests.

The use of natural progesterone has largely been led by women desperate for help with menopausal symptoms who have sought an alternative to HRT. There is a wealth of anecdotal evidence in its favour. I should say at this point that I tried it out of interest when I became fed-up with weight gain from conventional sequential HRT in the perimenopausal period. The hot flushes did improve and returned when I stopped taking it. The weight stayed, which makes me suspect it's metabolism and enjoyment of food that's the culprit, rather than the hormones. I'm now taking part in a trial, so I don't know whether I'm on the real stuff or a placebo (I am still asking 'Is it me or is it hot in here?' so, who knows?) There'll be more info when the book is revised in a year or so's time. It is significant, though, that many more clinical trials are beginning to be conducted.

Two trials going on at the moment in Britain are being carried out by Dr Adam Carey from the Reproductive Medicine Trust at the Chelsea and Westminster Hospital and Northwick Park Hospital. They are funded by one of the companies which imports the cream into Britain.

The first is a double-blind placebo-controlled trial to evaluate the effects of the cream on climacteric symptoms and the safety of the treatment. Approximately 180 post-menopausal women between 40 and 60 will be tested. Results are due late next year. The second is testing women at risk of osteoporosis who have chosen not to take oestrogen. Dr Carey says there is evidence *in vitro*, under laboratory conditions, that progesterone can stimulate bone-building, but there is not enough evidence yet to show whether it works in the human body. Results are expected in two years' time.

The National Osteoporosis Society says there is not enough evidence yet to recommend the use of natural progesterone creams to prevent osteoporosis. It is part-funding another study in Southampton, and results are expected in 2002.

Heart disease
Laboratory work has shown that progesterone has the ability to relax coronary artery muscle cells, but there is no evidence to suggest that it can actually help to prevent CHD.

SCEPTICISM

Overall, most doctors are still sceptical about natural progesterone and won't be convinced until properly formulated clinical trials give them the evidence they think is necessary for every drug. They are not convinced by Dr John Lee's evidence from clinical practice, which they would describe as 'bad science' without the academic rigour required. Dr Adam Carey, on the other hand, describes him as a 'good doctor who has pursued what he believes is best for women and treated them holistically'.

But even some of the anti-HRT alternative practitioners are not convinced either. Marilyn Glenville, a nutritional therapist and author of *Natural Alternatives to HRT*, says we may be jumping on the same bandwagon as we did with conventional HRT, looking to replace a 'deficiency' which may not need to be supplemented with a substance which may not be safe. She emphasises that the 'natural hormone' is no more natural than the plant-based 'natural' oestrogens used in HRT, and she says:

> There is nothing natural and nothing alternative about it. Surely the aim is to get our bodies back into balance naturally and to allow our bodies to do this themselves. By adding in any kind of direct hormone, we are never addressing the fundamental cause of the problem. If you stop the cream, you are back to square one: your body will not have become any healthier in the process.

PHYTO-OESTROGENS

Marilyn Glenville and Maryon Stewart, the other natural menopause guru and founder of the Women's Nutritional Advisory Service, are both fans of phyto-oestrogens, which they believe are the true 'natural' alternative to HRT as part of a balanced diet, combined with exercise.

WHAT ARE PHYTO-OESTROGENS?

Phyto-oestrogens (POs) are naturally occurring substances in food that have a hormone-like action in the body. They are similar in structure to the oestrogen produced by the body, but are only $\frac{1}{250}$th to $\frac{1}{1000}$th as potent.

The theory is that POs act as 'good' (for menopausal symptoms and long-term health promotion) as opposed to 'bad' (cancer-causing) oestrogens. In other words they are Nature's version of SERMs (selective oestrogen receptor modulators) discussed earlier (see p. 133). Maryon Stewart says:

POs are fast becoming known as great hormone regulators, in that they can both increase and decrease the levels of oestrogen in the body, depending upon the circumstances. When oestrogen is in oversupply in the body, as can occur prior to the menopause, POs play musical chairs with oestrogen in competition with the receptor sites within the cells. Some of the POs will inevitably displace oestrogen and, because they are many times weaker in their effect, they reduce the cancer- promoting effects of the hormone proper. POs also dilute the effects of environmental oestrogens (xenoestrogens) which can be even more harmful to the body than normal oestrogens. On the other hand, if you are producing too little oestrogen, for example at the time of the menopause and beyond, phyto-oestrogens can give levels a natural boost, thus helping to combat symptoms such as hot flushes and osteoporosis.

A lot of the positive evidence cited about phyto-oestrogens is linked to the observed differences between women in Western and some Asian countries. Japanese women, for instance, are far less likely to suffer from hot flushes at the menopause than their Western counterparts. They also have lower rates of breast cancer – one quarter of the incidence found in Britain and America – and a better survival rate. Yet, studies have shown that when they move to the West and adopt a Western diet and lifestyle, cancer rates mimic those found in the West in a very short period of time.

Animal studies have spurred scientists to look further into the effects of POs. In Australia it was found that sheep became infertile after grazing on large quantities of red clover. Cheetahs in captivity fed on high levels of POs also had reproductive failure and were found to have changes in their bodies similar to those in women taking the pill, but humans have not shown similar effects when eating moderate levels of POs.

WHERE ARE THEY FOUND?

Some 300 plants are thought to contain POs, but research is still needed to determine exactly how much. Almost all fruit, vegetables and cereals (grains such as rice, oats, barley and wheat), seeds and some herbs (including cinnamon, sage, red clover, hops, fennel and parsley) have some POs. In particular, soya beans, linseeds, chickpeas and lentils are the richest sources. The active ingredients are not hormones in themselves, but bacteria in the gut convert them into substances which have an oestrogen-like action.

The most talked-about group of POs are isoflavones. There are four important kinds:

- genistein
- daidzein
- biochanin A
- formononetin

Soya ranks highest for isoflavone content, and contains the largest concentrations of genistein and daidzein. Chickpeas, lentils, mung beans and aduki beans contain substantial levels of all four types of isoflavones.

Other classes of POs include:

- lignans – found in seeds, fruit and vegetables, but most of all concentrations are found in linseeds (flax seeds).
- coumestans – the main one is coumestrol and the richest food sources are mung bean sprouts and alfalfa sprouts.

It's estimated that the average Japanese woman's daily intake of isoflavones is between 20mg and 80mg per day, but American and British women generally consume less than 5mg.

Soya: the miracle food?

Soya is especially rich in POs and has been studied in detail. The soya bean is also one of the best plant sources of protein and is free from saturated fat, so it has a lot of general beneficial dietary potential. While soya products are staples in Asian countries, they have been eaten in the UK mainly by vegetarians.

The basic form of soya is dried soya beans. Fresh ones are harder to come by in this country than in Asian countires and the dried ones can take a long time to cook and taste rather bland on their own. They are best added to soups and casseroles.

Soya beans have many, more palatable, by-products:

- *Soya* milk, where the liquid is extracted from the soya bean and sold on its own or with added flavours, calcium or sweeteners. It can be used in the same way as cow's milk.
- *Tofu* – soya bean curd. This can be eaten on its own and is especially good steamed and served with a good-quality soy sauce, a little sesame oil, chopped coriander and spring onion.
- *Soya-flour* – extracted from soya beans. It can be used to substitute a third to a quarter of other flours in baking.
- *Soya flakes*, made from toasted dried soya beans. They can be added to cereals, biscuits and breads.
- *Soya nuts* can be bought and eaten as snacks.
- *Breads* containing soya and linseed are available in some health-food shops.
- *Miso* – a fermented soya-bean paste used heavily in Japanese cooking and Indonesian tempeh – a fermented soya-bean pâté.
- *Soy sauce* – a product of fermented soya beans. This is generally not consumed in large enough quantities to give isoflavone benefit.
- *TVP* – textured vegetable protein or soya mince. It can be used as a meat substitute and is common in pre-packaged vegetarian meals.
- *Dairy-free products* made from soya, including yogurts, drinks, desserts, cheese and soya cream.

Generally, the more processed the soya, the fewer isoflavones it contains – check the label or choose a traditional food if in doubt. Marilyn Glenville also says that in different forms of soy, the isoflavones are absorbed at different rates. The fermented products, such as miso and tempeh are especially good for absorption.

RECOMMENDATIONS ON EATING PHYTO-OESTROGENS

Marilyn Glenville says that as a guide, research has estimated that you should try to include 45mg of isoflavones each day in your diet. A typical serving is 55g (2oz) of tofu, or 600 ml (1 pint) of soya milk. Each contains 35–40mg of isoflavones.

Maryon Stewart points out that some soya milk and yogurt can contain relatively low levels of isoflavones and recommends one serving of soya protein per day on top – either half a mug of tofu, tempeh, TVP or soya beans.

Although there is a lot of interest in soya, it is important to see it in the context of a balanced diet. Far from being a miracle food, it can have adverse consequences when consumed in high quantities. It can, for example, lower the absorption of vitamins A, B, C and E, and can also reduce iron levels, which may be why oriental women balance it with seaweed, which is rich in iron. Marilyn Glenville says it is important to remember to eat other phyto-oestrogen-rich foods, such as chickpeas and lentils, and recommends a daily tablespoon of linseeds which can be sprinkled on cereal or in yogurt. A full range of POs is essential for balance.

Suzannah Olivier, author of *The Breast Cancer Prevention and Recovery Diet*, says it is important to take a varied diet of foods containing POs because some people can develop allergies to soya. She says it's probably a good idea to introduce soya into the diet slowly and give the body a chance to acclimatise over a couple of months. Unlike the Japanese, we are not used to consuming soya from childhood.

GENETIC MODIFICATION

Soya is also a prime target for genetically modified organisms (GMOs). I remember Linda McCartney's concerns about this when I interviewed her. Sir Paul spent millions of pounds after she died, searching all over the world for GMO-free soya in order to continue her vegetarian food business and had great difficulties finding sources that were GMO-free. Check the label if you have concerns. (There'll more information about diet and the use of soya and phyto-oestrogens in Chapter 7.)

THE DEBATES AROUND PHYTO-OESTROGENS

Ruth Lea of the Institute of Directors stopped her HRT after ten years when she concluded that it was not as beneficial as she had been led to believe. She was not at high risk of osteoporosis and found out herself that it only postpones bone loss for as long as you take it. She also researched the claims for prevention of heart disease and stroke and concluded that, again, there was very little epidemiological evidence to support them.

Lea's research on cervical cancer screening (see Chapter 3) convinced her that there was 'an epidemic of anxiety around women's health'. It made her 'a total sceptic about everything doctors do and say'. She became irritated by a doctor's assumption that her menopause, far from being a natural life event, was a deficiency. When we talked on the phone and I asked her whether she took anything now, in her early fifties, she laughed and rushed to her kitchen cupboard. She gave me an impressive list of supplements which we'll discuss in a moment (they include black cohosh, starflower and evening primrose oils, red clover, sage, dong quai, liquorice, glucosamine sulphate for her joints, garlic for the heart and cod liver oil) and listed the additions to her diet which she had begun after reading Marilyn Glenville's theories about phyto-oestrogens. She eats Yofu yogurt and takes Phytosoy as a supplement. She also eats lots of oily fish including mackerel, herring and tuna, and says she's never felt better.

Lesley Hilton, the medical journalist, on the other hand, took Menolife which she bought from the chemist, ordered Phytosoy by mail order and ate Linda Kearns' HRT cake. The whole lot was costing her £40 a month which she could ill afford and when she found there was no effect on her hot flushes and exhaustion she gave them all up.

Moyra Livesey of the Rylstone WI was reluctant to take HRT when her perimenopausal symptoms began. She had been to a meeting where the menopause was discussed and it was suggested that red clover and soya might be helpful for women who wanted to avoid conventional treatment. She says the red clover was very expensive, the Blackmore's Phytolife Plus (including calcium) was less so and she thinks that for about six months they did help. Then the hot sweats and daytime flushes started to become almost unbearable and her periods much heavier and erratic. In the end she plumped for HRT and has been fine.

PHYTO-OESTROGENS AND MENOPAUSAL SYMPTOMS

The reports of fewer hot flushes among women in Asian countries have been linked to the consumption of isoflavones. Studies have given mixed results. Some have shown a significant reduction in hot flushes by adding soya to the diet or using isoflavone supplements, but in general studies have been complicated by significant placebo effects. It seems that some women may benefit, but not all.

PHYTO-OESTROGENS AND LONG-TERM HEALTH ISSUES

Even when you're replacing hormones through your diet, there may be long-term health consequences to consider.

Breast cancer
It has been proposed that POs could reduce the risk of breast cancer from population studies which have linked the consumption of soya products on a regular basis to low rates of cancer.

The theory is that phyto-oestrogens fit into the oestrogen receptors in the breast and block the more potent and potentially damaging oestrogens. Genistein, one of the best studied isoflavones, has been shown to possess various anti-carcinogenic qualities, including being able to prevent the activation of the genes that cause cancer and also blocking the blood supply to cancerous tumours.

Fans of phyto-oestrogens quote studies using POs in animals which have shown reductions in the occurrence of cancer. In studies on rats, isoflavones have been shown to reduce tumour growth through their anti-oestrogenic properties and also their anti-oxidant effects.

Cell culture studies on human and animal tissue have indicated that POs can exert an anti-proliferative effect on breast tissue. In other words, they don't trigger significant cell multiplication. Studies in women diagnosed with breast cancer have shown they excrete lower levels of phyto-oestrogens in their urine (which is an indicator of dietary intake), compared with women without breast cancer.

Maryon Stewart concludes:

Current research shows that phyto-oestrogens are unlikely to be sufficient to inhibit the growth of mature, established breast-cancer cells. But it seems they will regulate the proliferation of the cancer cells, therefore having a chemoprotective effect. Research is young and much still remains to be learned about the influence of specific dietary constituents and cancer risk.

The medical profession as a whole urges caution, preferring not to make assumptions about a link between POs and a lower risk of breast cancer until further research is completed. The most recent study, carried out in Japan and published in 1999, was conducted by the Imperial Cancer Research Fund and looked at the consumption of soya foods and breast-cancer risk among Japanese women. It found no significant relationship between reported consumption of tofu or miso soup and breast-cancer risk.

There are also concerns that POs may have a negative effect on the breasts because they can be oestrogenic as well as anti-oestrogenic and the mechanisms by which they work in the body are not fully understood. Sensible levels of of POs are recommended and supplements containing high levels of isoflavones are not encouraged, especially for women who have had breast cancer.

Janet Balaskas, the founder of the Active Birth Movement, is only too aware of the current reservations about POs, but has taken advice from Marilyn Glenville, who believes they have been exaggerated. Janet became perimenopausal as she approached her fiftieth year – she's now 54 – and has found the whole transition from perimenopausal to post-menopausal woman extremely difficult. Her symptoms were horrible, she says, with hot flushes during the day and night sweats which woke her frequently at night, making her very tired the next day and her morale very low. She had never before been a depressive person. She describes it as being similar to the period when a new baby is very young and you feel in a state of permanent jet lag (she should know, she's had four children and worked with pregnant and newly delivered mothers for most of her adult life).

Janet was keen to take the dietary route to help her through and consulted Marilyn Glenville when she began to realise that her symptoms were an indication of the perimenopause. She had a hair mineral test which revealed what minerals her body needed (this is a disputed technique – some practitioners, including Dr Adam Carey, are not convinced it has validity; others swear by it) and she was given guidelines on eating phyto-oestrogens. She now includes soya products, nuts, seeds, tahini, whole grains, fresh fruit and lots of dark green vegetables in her diet. She also sees a homeopath for other forms of treatment.

Most significantly, she had a breast scan at the beginning of her perimenopause and found lots of benign fibrocystic lumps. She chose to have the scan and pay for it herself as her gynaecologist no longer recommends mammogram, believing the X-rays to be potentially harmful, and instead uses only an ultrasound scanner which is highly sensitive and can detect even the smallest abnormality. She gave up coffee, tea and alcohol (caffeine can make the cysts worse), followed the recommended PO diet and took Three Treasures Phytosoy and red clover. The cysts have, five years on, completely disappeared, which, she believes, is the result of following Glenville's guidance.

Janet does not dismiss the potential risk and agrees that women at this time of life face an incredible dilemma. If you do nothing, you can end up feeling quite dreadful and unable to carry out the necessary tasks, but she agrees there is no 'no-risk' option. The choices, she says, are very difficult and require a lot of thought and information, especially as the transition from peri- to post-menopause can take so long – in her case, five years. She has a busy working life, a partner and her youngest son is still only 12. It's a question, as with all the treatments on offer, of carefully balancing risks and benefits.

Osteoporosis

Again research is in its infancy, but has indicated some potentially promising results. It is thought that POs may:

- inhibit bone breakdown by osteoclasts
- enhance bone growth by boosting activity of osteoblasts and increasing the production of bone matrix proteins

- enhance the secretion of calcitonin, a natural thyroid hormone which prevents bone breakdown by inhibiting osteoclasts and allowing osteoblasts to build bone

Soya also contains other nutrients such as vitamin K, which may contribute as well to the preservation of bone. Even though protein is necessary for the maintenance of strong bones, it is thought that excess intake increases urinary excretion of calcium. It has been suggested that compared with animal protein, soya leads to less calcium being lost.

There is, however, a contrary view, mentioned earlier, which says that soya in high quantities can reduce the bio-availability of vitamins A, B, C and E and can reduce iron levels, which may be why Oriental women balance soya with iron-rich seaweed.

Animal research has already shown that a diet high in soya can improve bone, at least in rodents. Research on women published in the *American Journal of Clinical Nutrition* in 1998 was promising, but not dramatic. It followed 66 post-menopausal women for six months to see if soya protein containing various amounts of isoflavones would improve their bone density. A third received a high dose, a third a medium dose and the remainder were given a placebo. The control group had a 0.5 per cent decline in bone density, as is normal in untreated post-menopausal women. Those on medium dose had no gain or loss of bone. Women on the high dose showed no improvement in hip bone density, but their spine density increased by an average of 2.25 per cent.

Experts agree that no firm conclusions can be drawn without more research, but would say cautiously that a diet rich in POs may help to protect from osteoporosis, although other dietary elements such as calcium are also important, together with weight-bearing exercise (see Chapter 7).

Heart disease

This is perhaps the most well-established benefit of PO-rich food. In October 1999, the American Federal Drug Administration sanctioned the promotion of some soya products for cardiovascular protection. After reviewing an analysis of independent studies they agreed that consuming 25g (1oz) of soya protein daily as part of a diet already low in saturated fat may help to reduce the incidence of coronary heart disease. The research showed how eating soya protein regularly can lower overall cholesterol by an average of 9 per cent and lower the unhealthy LDL type of cholsterol by 13 per cent. Again, it is wise to be wary of overinflated claims made by the food industry as it is isoflavones that are most likely to be beneficial, although these may be lost in the production of pre-prepared foods.

The isoflavones have strong antioxidant properties and it is widely believed that foods rich in antioxidants (e.g. fruit and vegetables) may help to reduce risk from coronary heart disease. Soya is also a useful source of soluble fibre which can lower cholesterol levels.

PHYTO-OESTROGEN SUPPLEMENTS

Isoflavones, as we have gathered from our anecdotal evidence, are also available in supplement form. These are extracted either from soya or from red clover, which is a herb rich in all four isoflavones. There is an abundance of these supplements on the market, but there are concerns that taking the POs out of food may alter their effects. Maryon Stewart warns that the majority of supplements are not scientifically based and research indicates that they will not have the same protective effects as soya-based foods. Dr Helen Wiseman, a nutritional biochemist from King's College London, compares it with eating an apple, and says there may be something within the apple that makes the vitamin C work better – it's the same with POs.

Again, it would seem wise to take the advice of a properly trained nutritional expert before shelling out a load of money buying over-the-counter remedies. In her own practice at the Women's Nutritional Advisory Service (WNAS), Stewart does recommend an isoflavone-rich supplement, as Western women may find it hard to adapt their diet sufficiently. Marilyn Glenville believes that taking a supplement in the short term is a safe option while we adapt our diet to accommodate higher levels of soya and other sources of POs. She does, however, urge caution as regards taking them for a prolonged period as not enough is known about the long-term effects of high doses of what is acknowledged to be a powerful substance. The WNAS prescribes a red clover extract which has a standardised extract of 40mg of isoflavones. It has undergone trials at New York University School of Medicine and showed that menopausal women who took one tablet each day showed a reduction in the intensity and number of hot flushes and night sweats.

ATTITUDES OF THE MEDICAL PROFESSION

At a meeting of the North American Menopause Society in 2000 a third of the time was spent talking about phyto-oestrogens, which was regarded by a number of doctors attending the conference as a sea change from the usual atmosphere. The agenda in the past has been dictated by HRT.

Dr Yehudi Gordon is a consultant gynaecologist at St John and St Elizabeth Hospital in London and he has begun referring patients who have difficulty taking HRT to Marilyn Glenville for nutritional advice. She notices that there is more interest now from doctors than ever before and that a number of them are following Dr Gordon's lead.

He admits that he has a more 'integrated' approach than many of his colleagues, but believes that both doctors and patients are becoming increasingly aware that diet is important and that there is a relationship between what we put into our bodies and what we get out. He believes menopausal women should have a nutritional assessment, rather like a car would have an MOT, and says it's important to address dietary issues whether you're taking HRT or not.

Dr Joan Pitkin, the medical advisor to this book and one of the country's leading experts in the menopause, is also enthusiastic about the potential of POs, but she is not yet convinced they can do everything HRT can. She is looking forward to properly constituted clinical research to establish unequivocally whether or not there are fewer cases of breast cancer and fractures in women who have adopted this approach.

CAUTION

Even the publication *What Doctors Don't Tell You* urged caution in its August 2000 issue, in welcoming POs as a miracle cure without firmly establishing the nature of their effects on breast cancer, the result of introducing soya late in life, the effects of supplements versus food, and whether the Japanese have fewer symptoms of menopause or of breast cancer because of other dietary and lifestyle factors. Investigations into the effects of eating less fatty meat, more fish and vegetables and less processed food – all typical of the Japanese diet throughout life – are urged.

The journal concludes:

> *much of what women are told about phyto-oestrogens is intelligent guesswork. In reality we have no idea what will happen when we begin to dramatically change the ratios of exogenous (originating from outside) to endogenous (originating from inside) hormones in the body. No-one particularly wants to burst*

the bubble founded on an all-natural cure for the menopause. However, in our rush to embrace an alternative to HRT, we may also be threatening the health of women in ways we cannot forsee – the ultimate deception from a profession that promises 'safer alternatives'.

We can only hope that someone, somewhere will find the money to conduct this research. Paying more attention to what gives Japanese women an easier passage through the menopause and keeps their breast-cancer risk relatively low is precisely what Germaine Greer has called for and which was mentioned in Chapter 2. Let's find out what makes us well rather than what will cure us once we are sick.

HERBAL MEDICINE

As Ruth Lea made clear when she introduced me to her kitchen cabinet bursting with a barrage of herbal remedies, there are lots of products on the market that will claim to help with the menopause. In this section we're examining some of the most popular ones such as red clover (see Supplements on p. 202), dong quai, black cohosh, wild yam, sage, liquorice and ginseng. As we've already seen, lots of drugs, including those hormone replacement therapies which are not derived from mares' urine, come from plants, but these are single active ingredients, isolated and synthesised in the laboratory. Herbal drugs are extracts from the whole plant and contain many different constituents. The theory is that, like the apple analogy made earlier in relation to phyto-oestrogens in food, the many ingredients in the plant all balance each other and the key ones are made more or less powerful by the other substances present.

EVENING PRIMROSE OIL

Again, this is one of Ruth Lea's armoury of treatments and Gloria Hunniford takes it as she's convinced that, along with vitamins E and C, it is good for her skin. It is one of the richest sources of the omega-6 fatty acid called gamma linoleic acid (GLA). The body needs it for the production of prostaglandins which play an important role in vital processes, including fluid balance and the reproductive system.

There is very little research on the usefulness of evening primrose oil (EPO) during the menopause although one small study did compare the experiences of women taking two doses of 1000mg each per day with those taking a placebo and the oil proved to be better than the placebo at reducing night sweats, but had no effect on daytime hot flushes.

Some women may find it helps to reduce breast tenderness which can develop as a side-effect of HRT – it generally only occurs during the first few months of treatment and the oil can help get through this stage. A high dose is recommended for this purpose. One study showed that women who took 3g per day of EPO (which would deliver 240mg GLA) compared favourably with those given two drugs commonly prescribed for breast tenderness. There were fewer side-effects too. Diuretics and vitamin B6 have been shown to be no more effective than placebo for this condition.

If you are taking evening primrose oil for menopause and not for PMT, for which it is also said to be useful, you can get it on prescription, although this may cost more than buying it over the counter. If you buy it yourself, make sure the dose is high strength and has no other ingredients besides evening primrose oil. Lower doses are often mixed with other substances for PMT.

EPO is also said to be an anti-inflammatory and can help sufferers from arthritis. It is recommended for skin, hair and nails and may help with fluid retention and mood changes.

BLACK COHOSH

Generally, clinical evidence in relation to herbs is sparse, but one of the most widely used for menopause and best studied is black cohosh. It's botanical name is *Cimicifuga racemosa* and it is a large, woodland perennial, native to North America and a member of the buttercup family. American Indians boiled the root and called it 'squaw root' as it was used in childbirth and to ease the pain of menstruation. It's believed to contain phyto-oestrogens.

Black cohosh has been studied in Germany and found to be useful in alleviating menopausal symptoms such as hot flushes, night sweats and depression. Critics of the tests carried out so far, however, have said the evidence is based on poor science as most studies were carried out on small numbers of patients and were brief, uncontrolled and unrandomised and few defined the participants' hormonal status before treatment. Black cohosh was approved by the German authorities for use as a treatment for menopausal symptoms, but it should be noted that Germany has a long history of combining conventional and herbal medicine. It is neither approved or otherwise by Britain or the USA because neither country imposes strict testing requirements for efficacy and toxicity on herbal remedies which are classed as food supplements. This should perhaps be reviewed as we discover more about the potential ill effects on breast tissue of powerful POs.

In April 2000, the Harvard Women's Health Watch reviewed all the evidence on the herb so far and concluded: 'Because no long-term safety studies exist, black cohosh should not be taken for more than six months, and because manufacturers' preparations differ, it is best to follow the dosing directions on the label. Anyone considering black cohosh for menopausal symptoms should find the dearth of good clinical evidence sobering and should be cautious about taking the herb until it is better investigated.' Fortunately, that may be soon. The National Institute of Health recently gave the Unviersity of Illinois at Chicago a $7.9 million grant to study ten of the most popular herbal remedies, including black cohosh.

DONG QUAI

Dong quai has also been used by a number of the women I have spoken to, but often in combination with a number of other herbal, over-the-counter remedies, so it is difficult to assess whether their increased sense of wellbeing is due to any one preparation or a mega placebo effect! It has been used in Chinese medicine for 2000 years and is said to help numerous disorders including menstruation, menopause and symptoms due to 'deficient blood energy'.

I have only managed to uncover one study of the herb, published in 1997 and carried out in California as a double-blind, placebo-controlled randomised trial in 71 women. They found dong quai to be no better than placebo in relieving menopausal symptoms, nor did it have any side-effects such as oestrogen-like responses in the vagina or thickening of the endometrium.

Dr Marion Everitt of the Leeds NHS Menopause Clinic is dismissive of over-the-counter herbs like dong quai because of the lack of evidence that they are useful, because they cost money which women can often ill afford – especially if there is no benefit to be gained from them – because they appear in hugely different doses from different chemists or health food shops and because they can be dangerous. She reminds me of two cases of British women who died from taking Chinese herbs for eczema which were reported in the medical journal the *Lancet* in 1999. There is generally no quality control on herbal remedies and the *Lancet* referred to the fact that Chinese herbs have been found to contain aristolochic acid which causes damage to the kidneys and can be carcinogenic. In Belgium there have been 100 cases of kidney disease related to Chinese herbs.

GINGKO BILOBA

This is an extract from the leaves of the gingko biloba, the maidenhair tree, which is the oldest species of tree alive today. The extract contains numerous chemicals, including various flavonoids which are among the most active ingredients. In animal and laboratory experiments, gingko extracts appear to increase blood flow and neutralise oxygen-free radicals. Tests in mice and rats have revealed little toxicity. It's traditionally used in Chinese medicine and is said to be important in helping to maintain brain functions such as memory and concentration because it helps blood flow.

There have been some small research projects, notably one at Guildford University earlier this year, which seem to indicate some positive effects of gingko biloba on the short-term memory of healthy people. Other work suggests it has some use in memory impairment caused by dementia, suggesting it may have a role in slowing the progress of Alzheimer's Disease, but more research is needed to draw reliable conclusions.

There are question marks over the use of gingko biloba among the healthy. Harvard Men's Health Watch recently noted that it has become the third best-selling herb in the USA, to the tune of $300 million a year, even though there is very little evidence that it works. They also warned that it may produce an increased risk of bleeding in people taking aspirin and anti-coagulants.

GINSENG

Ginseng is derived from a root and has been used for centuries in Far Eastern medicine. Its effects are relatively well-studied. Ginsenoside compounds are said to be similar to the body's own stress-busting hormones. Ginseng is said to enhance the body's own immune system and its ability to handle stress. It's also said to strengthen the adrenal glands, to help to counter fatigue and to regulate hormones. A 1999 Swedish study found it slightly better for symptom relief than placebo, but they reported more positive results on depression and well-being. It is, though, a stimulant and you are advised to avoid it if you have high blood pressure. Personally, whenever I have tried it, it has made me sick, so I can't comment on whether it works or not.

LIQUORICE

Liquorice may be helpful for menopause symptoms and for stomach acid problems. Like some of the other herbs it should be used with caution if you have high blood pressure.

ST JOHN'S WORT

St John's wort (*Hypericum perforatum*) is the herbal remedy recommended by Hippocrates in Ancient Greece as a remedy for demonic possession, so I guess it would have fitted his perception of a menopausal woman! It's now widely used to treat mild to moderate depression, costing on average, £17.95 for a month's supply. It's not really known how it works. It has at least ten compounds that may contribute to its pharmacological effects, including flavonoids and xanthones.

Research published in the *British Medical Journal* in 1996 and in Germany in 1998 showed it was as effective as conventional treatments in boosting mood and had fewer side-effects, but there are cautions. It can react dangerously with other drugs including Warfarin, used for blood thinning, and tetracycline, which is a common antibiotic. Yet, like all other herbal preparations and despite its powerful pharmacological effects, it is not licensed as a drug in this country, but is sold as a food supplement. Edward Ernst, professor of Complementary Medicine at the University of Exeter, warns: 'In Germany it is a registered drug with standardised preparations. In the UK, the amount of St John's wort in any preparation can vary from 100 per cent to zero. Doctors know very little about it and what doses are needed.'

SAGE

Interesting work is now being done on sage as a treatment for hot flushes. A traditional remedy is to drink sage tea, made by steeping one teaspoon of garden sage in a cup of boiled water, then straining and sipping.

The tests are being carried out by Bioforce, a Scottish company which produces a sage tincture. The researchers believe that sage, like the other herbs mentioned and liquorice, is adaptogenic, which means it can boost levels of hormones which are too low or alternatively block the uptake of hormones if the body has produced too many. They believe that sage helps to block the mechanism described in earlier chapters which causes the hot flush. The current pilot trial involves 40 women and it is hoped that the numbers will be increased.

Note: There is some debate as to whether you should use sage if you suffer from high blood pressure.

SEEING A QUALIFIED HERBALIST

If you choose this route for yourself you should remember that it is generally agreed that those herbs that have powerful effects on the body can be dangerous as well as helpful and it is recommended that you see a qualified person to guide you. Self-prescribing goes against the grain of the way medical herbalists work. They treat each woman differently and take account of medical history, diet and lifestyle, as well as any other drugs you may be taking. They want to know what may inter-react with any herbs they prescribe. They may also feel it necessary to prescribe a number of herbs which will work well together for you.

The National Institute of Medical Herbalists (NIMH) tell me their members have to undergo a minimum of three years' training. Expect to pay £35 for the first consultation and less for follow-ups. Medicines will cost around £4 to £6 a week. Their information officer, Trudy Norris, tells me she has treated a number of women who have been unable or unwilling to take HRT. The majority have reported a reduction in unpleasant symptoms.

The NIMH are doing their own Menopause Audit as they are concerned that women who are vulnerable around this time may be putting themselves at risk through self-prescribing or wasting money on ineffective treatments. They do, however, have concerns about trials of individual herbs carried out under the same conditions as for drugs. They say that because they may use a number of herbs in treatment, testing single herbs or their individual constituents does not reflect practice. The *New England Journal of Medicine*, on the other hand, says, 'There cannot be two kinds of medicine, conventional and alternative. There is only medicine that has been adequately tested and medicine that has not – medicine that works and medicine that may or may not work.'

ACUPUNCTURE

Acupuncture can be used with other complementary therapies to try to correct hormone and energy imbalances during the menopause. Available patchily on the NHS, it's a branch of Chinese medicine in which needles are inserted through the skin at specific points on nerve or energy pathways called meridians. It's based on the principle that *chi* (energy) moves along these meridians and when blockages occur, pain or illness results. The needles stimulate points along the meridians to reduce or increase the energy flow and remove blackages. Only one person in my sample tried it for her menopause, Janet Balaskas, and found it had no effect.

HOMEOPATHY

Homeopathy is based on the theory of treating like with like and attempts to encourage the body's own healing mechanism by treating it with minute quantities of substances which would produce the same symptoms. Remedies can be bought over the counter but, like herbalism, homeopathy is not about treating symptoms with a blanket approach, but treating the whole person, taking into account all other influences. Practitioners take detailed individual histories and prescribe holistically.

There are currently five NHS homeopathic hospitals and a number of community-based and independent clinics where qualified homeopathic doctors work. Some GPs and primary health-care workers have also trained in homeopathy. You can often be referred for treatment by your GP.

There are around 2000 homeopathic remedies, but only about 40 are in common usage. Sceptics point to the lack of clinical trials to show how homeopathy works, although trials which have been conducted seem to show that it does work. Both Gloria Hunniford and Janet Balaskas have used homeopathy successfully during the menopause and beyond. When Gloria has a particularly heavy schedule she visits her homeopath to devise a programme to help her energy levels. When she broke her shoulder when she was 50 and it failed to mend she was threatened with a transplant of bone from her hip. She says homeopathic treatment helped her bone and tissue to mend and she didn't need the operation. Both emphasise the importance of seeing a qualified practitioner, whether on the NHS or privately.

AROMATHERAPY

Aromatherapy is one of the fastest growing of all complementary therapies, probably because it's such a pleasure to lie down for an hour or so and be pampered. Who could feel depressed with all that warm and caring attention?! It's a treatment that was familiar among the Ancient Greeks and Egyptians and was revived in the

1940s when a French chemist accidentally spilled some lavender onto a cut which healed without scarring.

There is an increasing crossover with conventional medicine as aromatherapy becomes a more common treatment in hospitals and hospices. A trial funded at Birmingham Women's Hospital was begun in 1999, but has not yet reported. Nevertheless, the treatment is said to be useful for depression, insomnia, and anxiety and is an aid to relaxation.

Camomile oil, in particular, is said to be a soothing, calming anti-depressant. Other oils thought to work as anti-depressants and relaxants are bergamot, clary sage, jasmine, lavender, neroli, sandalwood and ylang ylang.

HORMONAL EFFECTS

Aromatherapy oil is most commonly used as a massage oil or diluted in the bath. Many of the oils are said to have a hormonal action in that they affect the endocrine system. Basil and rosemary stimulate the adrenal cortex and geranium is thought to be especially useful as a general hormone balancer.

Other oils have oestrogenic properties in the form of phyto-oestrogens, but the substances behind these qualities are not well understood. Oils in this category include clary sage, fennel, star anise and tarragon. As with other similar substances with an oestrogenic action, care needs to be taken when using them.

HEAVY BLEEDING

Aromatherapy is often recommended to help to regulate the menstrual cycle and heavy bleeding, although some oils can stimulate bleeding. Cypress is thought to be helpful for heavy bleeding, but before taking it, discuss the problem first with a doctor or gynaecologist as the bleeding may be a symptom of fibroids or other problems. Cypress, geranium and rose are said to have a regulating effect. Rose is recommended as an overall good thing for the menopausal woman as it not only promotes a feel-good factor because of its smell, but is also said to act as an anti-depressant and aphrodisiac and is a good oil for nourishing older skins.

In the introduction to *Aromatherapy: an A-Z*, Patricia Davis, warns that if you are going to use them without the guidance of a trained therapist, you should buy essential oils that are as pure as possible and be suspicious of cheap ones – 'buy essential oils as you would buy fine wines'.

As with so many other complementary therapies, if you are going to use the treatment to help to ease menopausal symptoms, it is probably wise to see a trained therapist. The oils are far from benign and need to be used with care. Maggie Tisserand, who is an expert, has written 'Every woman's experience of menopause is different and the aromatherapist needs to take this into account when considering treatment.'

Oils to avoid if you have high blood pressure are bergamot, camomile, clary sage, cypress, pine, rose absolute, rosemary and thyme. Don't use bergamot, lemon, grapefruit, mandarin or orange if you are planning to sunbathe.

CONCLUSION

It's obvious that if a product is to have an effect, it must contain certain powerful ingredients, which may carry risks, just as more conventional medicines do. Again, don't be fooled by the words 'natural' or 'alternative'. Some of these products may be really helpful, but if in doubt, check it out with a reputable specialist in whichever field you choose.

And so we move on to the ideas which require a little hard work on your part – diet and exercise!

CHAPTER 7

DIET AND EXERCISE

Every ounce of good sense tells us that a healthy diet and plenty of exercise are more vital now than at any other time of life. Dr David Ashton, the author of *The Healthy Heart Handbook for Women*, tells me that he is concerned that exaggerated claims for the potentially protective effects against coronary heart disease of HRT, phyto-oestrogens or any other menopausal 'remedy' may lull us into a false sense of security and give us an excuse to ignore the hard facts. That CHD kills more of us than any other disease and that with a little bit of effort on the exercise front, giving up fags, reducing alchohol intake and adjusting the diet, we can vastly improve our chances of survival into old age with enough fitness and energy to tackle whatever we want to do with the rest of our lives.

All of which sounds very virtuous, but I don't want you to imagine that I'm sitting here lean and mean as I prepare to deliver a lecture. For breakfast this morning I had toast and real butter with caffeinated coffee and I'm planning a lamb roast with all the trimmings, apple pie and cream for dinner – no dietary adjustment there. Instead of getting up and going for a long walk first thing, I snuggled under the bedclothes to listen to *The Archers* omnibus and now I shall sit in front of the computer until it's too dark to go out. Then I'll have a glass or two of something to chill out, making my usual excuses to myself that dry white wine is really a non-alcoholic drink.

As you'll have observed from the picture on the front of the book, I am what the *Daily Mail* columnist, Linda Lee Potter, recently described as 'stately, a rather large lady'. If she'd been on her usual waspish form (in a recent interview I had berated her for being hurtful to the likes of Anne Diamond or Mo Mowlam), she would simply and quite truthfully have called me fat. One bit of good news is that, whilst it's obviously daft to be very overweight because of the potential strain on the heart, the old 'You can never be too rich or too thin' idea is also nonsense.

Excessive dieting deprives the body of essential nutrients and during and after the menopause we know that it's those of us who carry a bit of 'plumptitude' who suffer the least dramatic effects of the fall in oestrogen, because we are producing more of it naturally than our thinner sisters. So being just a leetle bit well covered is probably good for hot flushes and bone density. It's also useful for filling out wrinkles. Whoever saw an apple-cheeked granny looking like a prune? To a degree, then, it's OK to be in the Melba Wilson camp. Someone told her that giving up chocolate would help to cure her hot flushes. 'Frankly,' she said, 'I prefer the hot flushes.'

I know, though, I can't go on being cavalier in relation to my heart, circulation and general suppleness. I've got away with it thus far – to 50 – living by the St Augustine maxim, 'Give me chastity and continency, but not yet.' Even the most hedonistic among us know you can't continue to abuse the only body you've got and expect it to serve you well without a little care and attention and the occasional service. I remember being told by Anne Powell, who had a heart attack when she was only 36, that she had to adjust her lifestyle to survive. She changed her diet, started taking regular exercise and gave up smoking. The latter was achieved in hospital in the immediate aftermath of the coronary, but then, as she says, 'You can't smoke in an intensive care unit.' It seems a pity to wait until impending doom concentrates the mind.

So, let's assume that we all want to be good in bed rather than confined to one, as the novelist Rosie Thomas puts it, it's better to be entering the Peking to Paris motor challenge than a nursing home. Even Teresa Gorman, the biggest fan of HRT, confesses she also needs to take more care with her diet than she used to. Her mantra is simple: 'fat is fattening'. She eats no chips, crisps or processed food, drinks only skimmed milk, has alcohol in moderation – maybe one glass with a meal – eats lots of fresh fruit and veg and starts her day with bran, half a banana and half a fat-free yogurt. She likes a high-fibre diet because she believes it acts as a human scouring powder (see Fibre, below). Her regime, she says, has kept her in public life and out of the mental hospital and the divorce court.

Janet Balaskas, founder of the Active Birth Movement, is perhaps the most strict with her diet of any of the women I've spoken to. Working on the advice of her nutritionist she eats soya products, nuts, seeds, whole-grain products, fresh fruit and lots of dark green vegetables. She drinks no coffee, tea or alcohol and eats no red meat. When I asked her how her family (partner and 12-year-old son) react to sharing her diet she was uncompromising in her response. Her partner does still enjoy the occasional steak which he has to get from friends or at a restaurant, as she can't eat it any more. As for the rest of the time, 'I'm in charge of food around here, so they either eat what I cook or starve.' It is, of course, a generally healthy diet for any age group and is obviously of great benefit to her. She is beginning to understand, she explains, what is meant by 'post-menopausal zest'. Joan Bakewell enjoys the kind of varied diet she has always eaten and occasionally notices she's putting on a bit round the middle. She uses the Weightwatchers 'points' diet for short periods to reduce her waistine when necessary, but do be wary of faddy diets – a properly balanced diet should maintain a healthy weight. Now the lecture.

DIET

At the time of the menopause the metabolism begins to change and some eating habits that didn't visibly affect you as a younger woman may now show up in the waistline. Hence my conviction that it's metabolism, not HRT, that causes weight gain – perhaps because we're lulled into a false sense of security by the myth of HRT as a magic bullet against all ills. Whether you take HRT or not, you need to pay more attention to what you eat than ever before if you want to stay generally well and mobile without carrying too much flesh around.

Balance is important – you can have too much of a good thing, but you don't have to cut out everything that's naughty. As we've already seen, there's much interest in the Japanese diet and the fact that it's rich in phyto-oestrogens (see Chapter 6). But it is a carefully balanced diet. Soya consumed in high quanitities can lower the bio-availability of vitamins A, B, C, and E and can reduce iron levels, which, as we've seen, may be why Oriental women balance their soya intake with iron and vitamin-rich seaweed.

BASIC GUIDELINES

First, the principles of a balanced diet, which will be good for the whole family, but will also keep you fit and control some of your menopausal symptoms.

Eat a wide range of foods which you enjoy, but try to get them in the right proportions and, most important of all, try to eat more fruit and veg. Five portions or more a day are recommended, organic where possible. This includes fresh fruit juice and dried foods, but not starchy foods like potatoes – so chips don't count!

One way to sneak them in is to buy a juicer, which gobbles up a wide range of fruit and veg, but can mean you miss out on fibre (see below). You should try to eat a variety of types and colours each day. Fruit and vegetables are good because they are full of antioxidant nutrients (see below) and a wide range of vitamins and minerals. They provide tasty fibre in place of fat and also work towards reducing the risk of heart disease and cancer.

In any balanced diet, the main food groups you'll need to think about are as follows:

CARBOHYDRATES

Six or more servings a day are recommended, but make sure you fill up on the right type. There are two main types of carbohydrate. *Starches*, or complex carbohydrates, found in breads, rice, pasta, potatoes, cereals, grains and some vegetables and pulses, and sugars, or simple carbohydrates. These are described as 'intrinsic' when they are found in fruits and vegetables, 'extrinsic' when found in sugar, honey, fizzy drinks, cakes, biscuits and confectionery, and 'hidden' when they are in baked beans, pickles, breakfast cereals, pizzas, tinned meats and vegetables (see Sugar below).

It's the starchy complex carbohydrates and intrinsic sugars that should form the bulk of a healthy diet. Eat all types, but choose the unrefined ones where possible. These are found in brown rice, wholegrain bread and cereals, fresh fruit and veg and pulses, and contain plenty of nutrients, including fibre, vitamins, minerals and other phytochemicals (see below). Refined carbohydrates such as white rice, white pasta, white flour and white bread contain fewer of these elements, but can still be eaten.

Complex carbohydrates are important because they are rich in nutrients, but also because they help to maintain a steady blood sugar level. They can help to control the appetite and consequently weight, to lower raised blood fats and help to control, or even prevent, diabetes. They can make a big difference to how you feel emotionally and physically before, during and after the menopause. A healthy blood sugar level will enable the female hormones which circulate naturally to be fully utilised and help to avoid unpleasant symptoms. Ups and downs in blood sugar levels can be regulated by regular intake of complex carbohydrates and avoiding too much sugar and stimulants. Complex carbohydrates also reduce the amount of fat in the body and increase the amount of fibre in the diet.

FIBRE

This is now known more correctly as non-starch polysaccharide (NSP). There are two types of fibre: insoluble and soluble. Because they are found in differing amounts in foods, a full range of nuts and seeds, fruits, vegetables, pulses and grains is necessary. Both types of fibre are useful if you are watching your weight, because they aid digestion, increase your feeling of being full and remove toxins.

Insoluble fibre

The main function of insoluble fibre is as a bulking agent. It helps to prevent constipation and keeps the large intestine healthy. Wholegrain cereals and wholemeal bread are a good source. To correct constipation, you need to increase the intake of insoluble fibre, which can also reduce the likelihood of diseases of the colon.

Fibre is thought to reduce the risk of cancer by absorbing or transporting toxic substances from the body (as Teresa Gorman said – a kind of human scouring powder). A number of experts have also suggested that there may be a relationship between constipation and breast cancer. Fibre is thought to help to prevent breast cancer by speeding the excretion of excess oestrogen through the body.

Soluble fibre
Soluble fibre can help to reduce blood cholesterol levels. Oats, fruit, vegetables and pulses (beans, chick peas and lentils) are good sources.

Beware the bran
Most people do not need to eat bran-enriched food or sprinkle raw bran on cereals, etc. Unprocessed or raw bran contains phytic acid which can reduce mineral absorption. I mentioned this in the earlier section on osteoporosis. Excess bran can also tend to be an irritant and loosen the bowels too much.

To work fibre into your diet, eat a wholegrain breakfast cereal such as muesli or porridge, eat wholemeal bread and make a high-fibre soup with beans and vegetables.

FAT

Fat is often perceived as the dietary bogeyman and low-fat processed foods abound on the supermarket shelves. But cutting down on fat is far too simplistic because some fats are worse for health than others and some are abolutely essential to human health. Some fat in the diet is necessary simply because it's a dense source of energy – 9 calories per gram compared with 4g for both protein and carbohydrates. The main types of fat – good and bad – are described below.

Saturated fats
Saturated fats are the fats that solidify at room temperature and exist in high quantities in meats, milk, eggs, butter and cheese.

These are the bad ones because they tend to increase blood cholesterol and are associated with heart and circulatory diseases. Don't cut them out – for heaven's sake – I'd never make any of my favourite Nigel Slater recipes without butter; toast with marg is a criminal act; milk and cheese have other essential nutrients, as we've seen – and life without ever eating roast beef or fillet steak is definitely not worth living. Try to buy leaner cuts of meat, use olive oil, instead of lard for cooking, buy skimmed or semi-skimmed milk and low-fat cheeses and yogurts, grill or bake rather than fry and consume everything else sparingly.

Trans fats

Trans fats are also baddies because they may have an even more detrimental effect on cholesterol than ordinary saturated fats because they raise LDL (bad) and lower HDL (good). Only tiny amounts exist naturally in meat and dairy products, but commercial hydrogenation creates them. They are used in processed foods to prolong shelf life and improve texture. Limit your intake.

Avoid hard margarines and cooking fats, savoury snacks, and take-away foods such as fish and chips. Choose soft margarine labelled 'trans-free'.

Polyunsaturated fats (PUFAs)

These tend to have a liquid consistency at room temperature or lower and exist in vegetable oils (such as sunflower or walnut) and most nuts. They have a positive effect on health as long as they are consumed within sensible limits. A certain amount is needed because they contain essential fatty acids (EFAs) – omega-3 and omega-6.

These EFAs help the growth and repair of cells and tissues; they help the blood to thin; can reduce inflammation and pain in the joints; and help with PMS and menopausal symptoms. They are

also said to help to keep the skin healthy, to reduce water retention
and to keep the vagina, skin and hair moist.

Omega-6

Omega-6 oils are found in nuts, seeds and oils (preferably
unrefined), such as walnut, sesame and sunflower. One special type
is gamma-linolenic acid which may be manufactured in the body
from naturally occurring linolenic acid, but the process may not be
working efficiently. Supplements of evening primrose oil are often
recommended as a boost.

Omega-3

Omega-3 oils include EPA and DHA which are found in the
greatest quantities in oily fish such as mackerel, herring and
salmon. Linseed oil is another source. Our low levels of
consumption of oily fish mean these are the fats our diets are likely
to be deficient in. Studies have shown that a regular consumption
of oily fish reduces the risk of heart attack. However, Dr David
Ashton, the heart expert, says evidence would suggest that a
balance between the two families of PUFA might be more
important for health than the actual amounts in the diet. So, cook
your mackerel in sunflower oil!

Mono-unsaturated fats

Again, eaten at sensible levels, these, too, are good for you. They
tend to increase HDL cholesterol and reduce the harmful form,
LDL and triglycerides. Mono-unsaturated fats should form the
highest proportion of fat in the diet and are found in olive oil,
grapeseed oil and groundnut oil, and in olives, avocados, many
nuts, and hummus. It's the relatively high proportion of mono-
unsaturated fat that makes the Mediterranean diet so much
healthier than our traditional diet.

Don't forget that Teresa Gorman is right when she says fat

makes fat. If you eat more than you can burn off in energy you will put on weight, whatever type of fat you consume. Obesity unquestionably puts extra strain on the heart and in post-menopausal women there may be a connection between being overweight and breast cancer. We've already discussed how fatter women continue to produce more oestrogen after the menopause.

PROTEIN

Protein is important for crucial bodily functions, but we don't need huge amounts. Large portions of protein can put a strain on some of the body's processes and use up energy in digestion. Lots of us do eat more than the recommended amounts and cutting down allows more calories to come from complex carbohydrates, some of which are, of course, proteins as well, such as pulses.

The best policy is to vary your protein sources. You should eat some meat and dairy for the B vitamins, iron and zinc they provide, but you should mix them with fish, soya, nuts and pulses to get the widest range of vitamins, minerals, phyto-oestrogens and essential fats. Poultry is generally lower in harmful fats and calories than red meat.

Excess animal protein in particular can lead to loss of calcium and have a detrimental effect on kidney function. Links between animal protein and breast cancer are not proven, but the charred and burnt bits from barbecued, chargrilled and barbecued meat contain substances which have been said to be potentially carcinogenic. Similar questions have been raised over nitrates and nitrites used in processed and smoked meats. Don't forget to balance your meat consumption with plenty of protective anti-oxidants from vegetables. The nutritionist Marilyn Glenville would go so far as to suggest cutting out red meat and reducing dairy products during the menopause and, as I mentioned earlier, Janet Balaskas, following her advice, feels wonderful.

SUGAR

The average woman consumes 90g (3oz–4oz) of sugar per day, which accounts for 20 per cent of total calories. Ideally, in older women seeking to preserve youthful energy levels (and perhaps looks) this intake should be halved for more nutritious and lower-calorie foods. As we approach the menopause we need fewer calories, but more nutrients, so we need to reduce foods that lack value and destroy the nutrients we have consumed. Sugar is the primary culprit.

The extrinsic refined sugars that appear in sweet foods such as cakes, biscuits and confectionery are the worst problem. They cause tooth decay, are low in essential nutrients, but high in calories and because we learn to crave them for an energy rush, they can cause unstable blood sugar levels (see Complex Carbohydrates).

In her book *Menopause Without Medicine*, the complementary medicine expert Linda Ojeda says:

> *Sugar significantly alters the levels of several hormones as they attempt to maintain a chemical balance within the body. The pancreas, liver and adrenal glands are all overstimulated by fluctuation in blood sugar levels. While our bodies can handle blood sugar highs in our youthful years, the day of reckoning comes when our systems lose their resilience. For menopausal women, symptoms of this change may be related to the inability of the worn-out adrenal glands to take over oestrogen production as the ovaries decline. When the glands are strong and healthy they are much more capable of secreting the amounts of oestrogen needed to prevent dramatic hormonal fluctuations which are related to menopausal symptoms.*

Linda Ojeda suggests that sweet foods can trigger hot flushes (though Melba Wilson, of course, says she prefers hot flushes to giving up chocolate). You can limit intake by trying to phase out sugar in tea and coffee, avoiding fizzy drinks and replacing some of the sweets, cakes and biscuits with fruit. Instead of using chemical sweeteners you might use small amounts of more natural sugars such as honey and re-educating your taste buds to appreciate sweetness in fruit and vegetables.

SALT

As with sugar, most of us consume far too much salt – up to 9g a day, when we should be aiming for 6g. It's not just the salt on the table that contributes to consumption, but the high levels in processed foods such as baked beans, sauces, savoury snacks and even breakfast cereals. High salt intake can lead to high blood pressure and heart disease. It can also stimulate water retention and bloating and lead to calcium being lost. It is possible to re-educate the body to enjoy less salty food by cutting down gradually. Try natural sea salt – it has more flavour and aroma, so you will probably use less.

PHYTO-OESTROGENS

This topic was covered extensively in Chapter 6 and our diet plan later in this chapter will include foods which are rich in phyto-oestrogens. You may also have heard of Linda Kearns' menopause cake which is now very popular as a source of phyto-oestrogen. Linda was actually discovered by one of the contributors to this book, the medical journalist, Lesley Hilton. Linda was unhappy on HRT. She had always been interested in diet and had been a wholefood eater all her life. When she discovered that soya and linseed oil are rich in phyto-oestrogens she made a flapjack-style cake for herself and friends and had encouraging results. The cake is now a major commercial enterprise and a month's supply of ten cakes costs £22.50. I've tried it and found it a bit like eating sticky sawdust, but you pays your money and makes your choice.

DRINKS

It's important to keep your fluid intake up during the menopause, to prevent dehydration during all those horrid hot flushes and night sweats. But make sure you're drinking the right type of fluids, as some may make you feel worse, rather than better.

Tea and coffee

Coffee contains three stimulants – caffeine, theobromine and theophylline. These all act on the central nervous system and can overstimulate the adrenal glands, causing anxiety, insomnia and shakiness. They are also dehydrating and have to be detoxified through the liver. Coffee is thought to have a negative impact on the absorption of nutrients from food and a high caffeine intake can affect calcium absorption by encouraging excretion. A high level of caffeine consumption has been linked to breast pain and benign fibrocystic breast disease. Cutting it out completely can help, as Janet Balaskas found.

If you are a real coffee addict, as I am, it's apparently better to wean yourself off it slowly as going cold turkey can bring on headaches, drowsiness and the shakes (and miserable mornings without that delicious fragrance filling the kitchen and that first delicious kick – I shan't be giving it up, but perhaps one cup, rather than six, will suffice.)

I'm delighted to report that decaffeinated coffee – the ultimate wimp's drink – is not really a help. There is less caffeine, but it has been through a chemical process and contains theobromine and theophylline. It can still cause breast pain.

Tea does not contain as much caffeine per cup as coffee, but can still lead to the loss of minerals and other nutrients. Tannin in black tea has a similar effect and, in my case, has the same influence that high tannin red wine has on my stomach – it makes me sick. Some teas, especially green tea, have protective benefits in the form of antioxidants which can help to protect against cancer and heart disease. It's also pretty gentle on the stomach. Herbal teas, which have no caffeine, can be a good way to moderate intake of the other more common hot drinks.

Alcohol

No, I'm not going to tell you to quit, as what's the point of getting through the menopause without the occasional tipple? Death would be a welcome release. Moderation is the key. The government recommends that women should drink no more than 21 units per week. One unit is half a pint of average-strength beer, a standard measure of spirits or a small glass of wine. For those of you who can easily knock back a bottle after work or over lunch with a gang of mates, a 75cl bottle of wine with an alcohol content of 14 per cent contains 10.5 units. That's half your weekly ration!

Alcohol can trigger hot flushes and deplete the body's essential nutrients, including those which are important for bones. It's also a source of empty, weight-slapping-on calories.

Dr David Ashton, the heart expert, puts his safe drinking limits for women at 14 units per week, including two or three days without any alcohol and a maximum of 5 units on any one day. A small amount of alcohol for menopausal women is a good thing in that it can help us to relax and be sociable, but he says there is no evidence that wine is better for the heart than other alcoholic drinks. Recent research suggests that beer has benefits too, although there are some experts who say red wine is the healthiest alcoholic drink.

Dr Susan Love and Suzannah Olivier are even more cautious, as they are convinced there may be a small link between alcohol and breast cancer. The theory is that alcohol boosts the amount of oestrogen in the blood. Both of them recommend only three glasses a week of your choice of alcholic beverage. Suzannah Olivier points out that you can get the antioxidant effects of red wine by drinking red grape juice (boring!)

Water

Drink plenty. As we get older we need more fluid. Drinking enough helps the kidneys to work well and rid us of toxins. Between one and two litres a day is recommended. Water in coffee or black tea is not included as they have dehydrating effects. If you don't drink enough water you may suffer from headaches, poor concentration and constipation. During the perimenopause, water is especially important as heavy bleeding and sweating mean we lose a lot of fluid.

Mineral water contains traces of important minerals for the bones, mainly calcium and magnesium, but, if you suffer from high blood pressure or heart disease, you should avoid those with a high sodium content. Water is also good for the skin, which dries out as you age. Skin that is well hydrated from the inside will survive better.

EATING TO HELP TO PREVENT HEART DISEASE AND CANCER

As we've already seen LDL – the 'bad' form of cholesterol – has a role in the furring of the arteries and can contribute to heart disease. So it's a good idea to reduce intake of foods which cause the liver to manufacture more LDL. These include all foods high in saturated fat such as fatty meat and full-fat dairy produce. Trans fats (see above) are also dangerous when taken in significant quantities and are found in a number of commercial margarines and other foods. Check labels carefully and watch out for saturated fats in cakes and biscuits.

Foods that contain cholesterol have less of a damaging effect than saturated fats, but will contribute to cholesterol levels in the body if eaten in significant quantities, so be wary of too much offal, eggs, shellfish, meat and dairy products (but no need to give up the shellfish altogether!).

The 'good' cholesterol, HDL, can be reduced by certain foods, including trans fats and too much polyunsaturated fat – so butter, used in moderation, is probably better than some of the margarines.

Some foods will lower LDL, the 'bad' cholesterol. Poly-unsaturates which are high in linolenic acid such as corn and sunflower oil are included in this group, as are mono-unsaturates such as olive and rapeseed oils. Mono-unsaturates are obviously generally better as they lower LDL without depleting HDL. Garlic will help to lower LDL as will soya beans and milk, fibre found in oats, pulses and most fruits and vegetables. Oily fish such as salmon, mackerel and herring contain omega-3 fatty acids which help to prevent blood clots and can slightly lower cholesterol. And the really good news is that it's generally agreed that one glass of beer or wine (only one, mind, and that's glass, not bottle!) most nights of the week may increase HDL.

ANTIOXIDANTS

The UK's National Heart Forum recommends that five varied portions of fruit and vegetables, lightly cooked or raw and including a range of colours, each day may reduce heart disease by up to 20 per cent. Fruit and vegetables are the primary dietary sources of antioxidants – vitamins, minerals and phytochemicals which prevent oxidisation of the blood. Surplus LDL needs to be oxidised to become dangerous, so a diet rich in antioxidants can help to prevent the furring up of arteries. Antioxidants are also said to be the most important vitamins for women who are ageing and are often said to have 'anti-ageing' properties. Gloria Hunniford is certainly a good advert for them – her skin and hair glow with life and she takes a particularly high dose of vitamin C – 1000mg. She is careful, however, to point out that she takes all her supplements on the advice of a qualified practitioner.

The main antioxidants are vitamins C, E, and beta carotene (the plant form of vitamin A found in carrots and sweet potatoes), a number of phytochemicals (see below) and the mineral selenium. They are said to boost the immune system, help to protect against cancer and heart disease and to promote healthy skin and bones. Vitamin A is good for vision, Vitamin E is said to help hot flushes, and nuts, seeds, some cereals and vegetable oils are good sources of vitamin E. Vitamin C is found most plentifully in rosehips, guava, chili peppers and capsicum. It's in most green vegtables, including lightly boiled sprouts and in kiwi, citrus fruits and blackcurrants.

Phytochemicals
Scientists are taking an increasing interest in this group of compounds found in foods which have antioxidant properties. Although there are many different types of phytochemicals, they can be broadly grouped into three main categories: flavonoids, bioflavonoids and carotenoids.

- *Flavonoids* are found in tea (green tea is thought to be especially useful), red wine and a number of fruits and vegetables. Early research suggests they may have a role in preventing cancers.
- *Bioflavonoids* are closely associated with vitamin C and are found especially in citrus fruits. A recent large study of middle-aged men found that there was a three-and-a-half times greater risk of heart attack in those who were deficient in vitamin C. They are also thought to help to strengthen the blood capillaries, possibly lessening hot flushes, and to preserve the collagen in bones and skin.
- *Carotenoids* include the orange pigment (beta carotene) found in carrots. Lycopene belongs to this family and is attracting a lot of scientific interest because of its anti-carcinogenic properties. It's also thought that an adequate intake of lycopene can reduce the incidence of heart attacks by up to 50 per cent. It's the red

pigment found in tomatoes (including tinned, ketchup and ready-made pasta sauces), red grapefruit and watermelon. Epidemiological research in Canada has shown that women with breast cancer eat fewer tomatoes and have lower levels of lycopene than healthier women. The British Nutrition Foundation is a little more cautious as there have so far been no placebo-controlled clinical trials in humans, which perhaps makes it premature to make such claims with absolute certainty, but a chilli con carne or spaghetti bolognese with low-fat organic mince, olive oil for cooking and a couple of tins of tomatoes chucked in can't do much harm, can it?

Another carotenoid with possible anti-carcinogenic properties is lutein, found in dark green leafy vegetables, such as broccoli, blackcurrants and potatoes. Other types appear in mangoes, red peppers, pumpkins, squashes and mushrooms.

The British Nutrition Foundation says the best advice at present is a plant-based diet with a wide variety of fruit and vegetables, including tomatoes and other sources of lycopene. Which is just what your mother has always told you – eat up your fruit and veg.

Selenium

Selenium is a trace element that is currently receiving a lot of interest in the press, touted as a miracle substance with a role in the prevention of all kinds of diseases as diverse as infertility (not a problem for our age group!), dementia, low thyroid function and even AIDS.

The body needs only tiny amounts of trace minerals, but selenium, it seems, can have a profound effect. It's an antioxidant and has been shown to protect against heart disease and some cancers. It's also said to slow down the premature ageing process. In one large study recently carried out in the US, selenium supplements of 200mcg per day were associated with up to 52 per cent fewer deaths from cancer of the lung, prostate and colon. Deficiency may increase the risk of these diseases. It's also been shown to help to reduce the pain of rheumatoid arthritis.

Selenium comes from plants or plant-eating animals and the amount that we eat depends on how much there is in the soil. In Britain content is low, whereas in the US it's high, so we need to take more care to ensure that we are getting enough. Brazil nuts are a very rich source of selenium – Jo Wagerman, who has adjusted her diet to include as little fat as possible except on the Sabbath when she eats whatever she likes – includes three brazil nuts in her daily regime. They contain on average 1530mcg of selenium per 100g. Other mixed nuts and raisins are the next most selenium-rich foods, containing 170mcg per 100g. Fish, seeds and offal also contain it, but in much lower amounts. It's not a good idea to take too much selenium – up to 1000mcg a day should be OK – as it can be toxic when taken in excess and cause nerve disorder and hair loss.

EATING FOR HEALTHY BONES

Calcium is a significant part of our bone mass, but getting enough is only part of the story for the prevention of osteoporosis (see other nutrients and exercise later).

The National Osteoporosis Society (NOS) recommends that women aged 20 to 45 have a daily intake of 1000mg of calcium per day. For women taking HRT who are over 45 the same amount should sufice, but for women over 45 who are not taking HRT they recommend 1500mg.

CALCIUM IN THE DIET

If you eat well, you should get enough calcium through food. Most people associate only milk and other dairy products with calcium, but it's also present in non-dairy foods such as:

- Beans – soya beans and others (tofu is a good source).
- Nuts – almonds and hazelnuts.
- Vegetables – green, leafy vegetables are a modest source of calcium, including spinach, kale, bok choi and broccoli.
- Fruits – dried figs, apricots and raisins have small amounts of calcium.
- Fish – the only animal protein which provides calcium, and then only if the bones are consumed, so whitebait or tinned sardines are useful.
- Grains and sesame seeds – grains only have a small amount, but sesame seeds are a good source. A bowl of muesli is an easy way of getting a reasonable dose.

You can also buy calcium-enriched cereals, soya milk and orange juice. If you don't like milk, try to sneak some calcium into the diet via cheesy pasta dishes or foods such as ice cream or hot chocolate. There has been some discussion of a possible link between milk and dairy products and cancer. Professor Jane Plant is a geochemist who believes she helped to cure her own breast cancer by cutting out dairy foods. Most doctors and specialists in the field have refuted her claims completely and say there is no sound scientific evidence of a link at all. If you are lactose intolerant or vegan make sure you eat plenty of vegetables and beans.

Note: Fruit gums and white chocolate are good sources of calcium, but absolutely useless for anything else.

THE CALCIUM PARADOX

Contrary to what many people believe, a high calcium intake does not necessarily result in high bone density or prevention of bone loss. Some populations have a low intake of calcium, but also a low rate of osteoporosis and the scientific research has given no clear answers as to why this should be the case. A popular theory is that too much dietary protein, specifically animal protein, may affect the body's ability to absorb calcium and instead it is excreted in the urine. The Inuit population of North Alaska fits this pattern. They consume large amounts of calcium, mainly through fish bones, but have one of the highest rates of osteoporosis in the world, thought to be because of the high protein content of their diet. Another study found that women who consume five or more servings of red meat a week had a significantly higher risk of forearm fracture than those who had it only once a week. So, it's probably a good idea to limit your consumption of animal protein, especially beef, lamb, pork or venison and replace it with fish, chicken or plant proteins on a number of days a week.

There are other substances which may inhibit calcium absorption. Salt taken in excess can have this effect. Nutritionists recommend a maximum of 6g a day for an adult, but the UK average, 9g, is already too high. Watch out for salt content in crisps, nuts and processed foods. Caffeine, too, may affect absorption because it's a diuretic, so you may want to limit coffee and tea if you have other risk factors for osteoporosis.

Phytic acid, found in bran and the seed coats of beans and grains, may also affect calcium absorption. Too much fibre in general means that food speeds through the intestines and there is not enough time to absorb the calcium. In *Strong Women, Strong Bones* Miriam Nelson concludes: 'These problems are unlikely to arise if you get your fibre from food. But unless your doctor has told you to add fibre – for example, by sprinkling bran on breakfast cereals – it's best not to, because you can get too much. Rather than adding bran to ease constipation, try to eat plenty of high-fibre foods, drink lots of water and exercise' (see Fibre on p. 221).

Fizzy drinks contain phosphoric acid as a preservative. This can lead to an excess of phosphorus in the blood and stimulate bone breakdown. The NOS says there is no hard evidence to show a detrimental effect on bone health, but you may want to cut down on them.

VITAMIN D

Vitamin D is vital to aid the absorption of calcium and it helps the process by which calcium turns into bone. In studies of fractures and calcium supplements, the only ones which really demonstrate a reduction in fractures are those in which calcium is consumed in combination with vitamin D. As we get older we need more vitamin D than younger people: elderly people in nursing homes are especially at risk of bone fracture as they tend to have a poorer diet and don't go out in the sun.

Most of us should get enough vitamin D by eating the foods suggested above and enjoying an active, outdoor lifestyle. If not, supplementation is a good idea.

MAGNESIUM

We are learning more about magnesium, one of the minerals which make up bone and important for other chemical reactions in the body. A deficiency in magnesium is increasingly seen as a risk factor for osteoporosis, since magnesium is needed for calcium to be properly absorbed. A diet rich in fruits, vegetables and whole grains should provide enough without supplementation.

OTHER MINERALS AND VITAMINS FOR BONES

There are a number of less well known minerals and vitamins which may play a crucial role in bone health. Studies are limited and more research is needed.

Potassium

Potassium, which is present in oranges and bananas, is one of the nutrients with proven benefits for bone health, although there is no research supporting the use of potassium supplements for bone.

Boron, copper, zinc, manganese and essential fatty acids
Boron, copper, zinc, manganese and essential fatty acids (EFAs) are all important for bone health. The magazine *What Doctors Don't Tell You* recently described boron as the forgotten mineral, and quoted a study which found women who took 3mg of boron daily decreased the amount of calcium lost in the urine, while increasing their oestrogen levels. Boron is found in apples, pears, grapes, nuts, leafy vegetables and most dairy products; copper in nuts, seeds, fruit, beans, sunflower oil, mushrooms and crab; and manganese in nuts, seeds and meat. The EFA omega-3 is found in oily fish, linseed oil, soya beans and walnuts; and omega-6 is in sunflower oil, sesame oil, eggs, turkey and evening primrose oil. For sources of zinc, see p. 242.

Vitamin K
Vitamin K plays a part in normal fracture healing and circulating levels of the vitamin have been found to be low in people with osteoporosis. Its sources are broccoli, cauliflower, soya beans and dark green leafy vegetables.

WHAT ABOUT CALCIUM SUPPLEMENTS?

As with the general needs of the body, it's important to look carefully at your diet before deciding whether calcium supplements are necessary. Also, consider factors which may be calcium-depletors such as smoking, drinking and lack of exercise. If you have low bone density or are at risk from osteoporosis, you may want to discuss supplements with a nutritionist, though bear in mind that it's much easier to overdo the consumption of any nutrient with tablets than it is with food. As we've already mentioned, excess calcium can interefere with absorption of other essentials such as iron or zinc and calcium itself is much more readily absorbed from food than from pills.

In *Strong Women, Strong Bones* Miriam Nelson quotes a friend of hers who went to the doctor for a check-up and discussed osteoporosis with her. 'She questioned me about my diet and told me I should be getting more calcium. I'd been reading about suppements and knew bioavailability was an issue. So I asked if there was a brand of calcium supplements available in liquid form with natural sugars. She said, "Yes, it's called milk!".'

Nelson recommends only two forms of calcium supplement (having worked out in advance how much extra you need, based on your diet). These are:

Calcium carbonate

Most supply around 200mg to 500mg per pill. As they require acid to dissolve it's recommended that they are taken at mealtimes when the stomach excretes the acid in greater quantities.

Calcium citrate

New evidence suggests this may be easier to absorb than other forms of calcium. Becasue it contains acid it can be absorbed at other times when you are not eating. It's usually more costly than calcium carbonate and usually contains only 200mg to 300mg of calcium, so you may need to take more pills.

Nelson suggests avoiding calcium phosphate, as we generally get plenty of phosphorus from the diet and it can interfere with calcium metabolism. Calcium glutamate and lactate supplements generally contain less calcium than the ones she recommends. She warns against supplements made from oyster shells or bonemeal because in the past some have been found to contain toxic substances, such as lead. She also says don't pay extra for 'chelated' calcium supplements as there's no evidence that they are in any way superior.

You may get mild indigestion, bloating, constipation or loose bowels from calcium supplements. To minimise the problems, spread consumption through the day and if you take only one tablet have it at night to give more time for digestion. Nelson suggests the 'vinegar test'. Put one tablet in a cup of vinegar and stir every five minutes. If the tablet hasn't disintegrated within 30 minutes, it won't dissolve in your stomach either. Switch to another supplement and throw away the vinegar after the test.

Finally, be wary of overdosing. More than 2000mg (2g) a day can lead to kidney stones and other problems.

OTHER VITAMIN AND MINERAL NEEDS AT THE MENOPAUSE

B VITAMINS

This is a group of vitamins – B1, B2, B3, B6 and B12 – which work together and are essential for growth and the proper development of a healthy nervous system. They aid body maintenance, food digestion and metabolism. Some clinical studies have shown that a deficiency in B vitamins can contribute to post-menopausal anxiety and irritability. B6 and B12, together with folic acid – folate – are also important for protection against heart disease as they may lower levels of a substance called homocysteine, which is broken down from dietary protein. Forty-seven per cent of British women are said to be deficient in folic acid.

All the B vitamins and folic acid are readily available in a well-balanced diet, particularly in leafy green vegetables such as spinach and broccoli, whole-grain breads and cereals, rice, nuts, milk, eggs, cheese, poultry, liver, fish, other meats, berries, potatoes, citrus fruits and juices. Some foods have folic acid added to them and have a Folic Acid Mark. In his *Healthy Heart Handbook for Women* Dr David Ashton says there is probably little advantage in taking supplements if your diet is rich in these foods, but they could be necessary if you think your diet is inadequate. In which case he recommends asking a pharmacist for advice about what supplements to take.

Vitamin D

Vitamin D is crucial to aid absorption of calcium (see page 237) and there is some evidence to suggest it may play a role in preventing breast cancer. It's found in the skin and 15 minutes in the sun each day without a sun block would provide all the body needs, but unfortunately you may risk skin cancer if the sun is very hot. Studies have shown that women living in Florida are never short of vitamin D, but those in Boston are. A good daily walk, summer and winter, not at high noon should help. Vitamin D is hard to find in food, although it does appear in fatty fish such as tuna, mackerel and salmon, and in liver and eggs. Mushrooms such as shiitake and morels have vitamin D and some cereals and milk have it added. If you do decide to take a supplement – and it can be helpful if you live in a gloomy climate like ours – don't take more than 10 mcg a day, as too high a dose (up to 50mcg) can cause kidney damage by causing excess calcium to be deposited in the organs.

Iron

Iron deficiency can be a problem for women with heavy periods. After the menopause, once periods have stopped, iron requirements are reduced, but in the perimenopause, when bleeding can be more frequent and more profuse than usual you may become anaemic, which can cause tiredness. You may need to consider supplements or boost your iron-rich foods which include offal and red meats, dark green vegetables, pulses and wholegrains, nuts and seeds and fortified breakfast cererals.

ZINC

Zinc is needed for adequate immune function and it helps to keep the skin healthy. It's also said to give a fillip to a flagging libido! The best places to find it are in oysters – which is presumably why they got their reputation as an aphrodisiac – crab, lamb, liver, steak, garlic, ginger root, nuts and seeds.

TO SUPPLEMENT OR NOT?

Opinion on supplements varies enormously. Everyone agrees that vitamin and mineral supplements are really no substitute for a healthy, balanced diet. Some believe such a diet provides everything we need as we grow older; others will argue that even a well-balanced diet cannot provide optimum nutrition, because intensive farming, food processing, storage, transport and environmental pollution inevitably deplete the food we eat.

Equally, some specialists will say it's impossible for the body to benefit from vitamins and minerals in the most perfect diet if we subject it to the other pressures of modern life such as smoking, drinking, medicines, excess sugar and salt, caffeine and the cooking process itself. And, while the menopause is not a disease in itself, ageing in general puts demands on the body and our bodies become less efficient at absorbing the necessary vitamins and minerals.

In the United States, anti-ageing supplements and medicines are huge business. At the American Academy of Anti-Ageing Medicine a barrage of treatments is on offer, including B12 injections, vitamins, enzymes, omega-3 oils, HRT, the hormone DHEA, whose levels soar when the body is most healthy, testosterone, melatonin and even human growth hormone (HGH). One practitioner decribes hormone replacement as 'most effective when you replace everything. It should be a symphony.' One woman of 55 takes 85 pills a day, plus a shot of HGH and says she feels marvellous. I suspect she rattles.

Endocrinologists in the States are sceptical about these costly treatments as no scientific studies have proved their efficacy and there may be risks involved. The primary concerns are that testosterone supplementation may be connected with prostate cancer in men and we've already discussed the potential risks of HRT for women. The cautious say anti-ageing progammes may be OK for an 80-year-old who's trying to buy a few more good years, but a healthy 50-year-old with 20, 30 or even 40 years left should treat them with caution. Thomas Perls, chief of Gerontology at Beth Israel in Boston says, 'I think these anti-ageing guys are hucksters and snake oil salesman. They paint a very grim picture of old age that doesn't match the reality. The retirement years can be a wonderful time if you take care of yourself.'

There are lots of multivitamin and mineral supplements on the market and some claim to be specially formulated for menopausal women's general health, menopausal symptoms and protection from osteoporosis. Dr Adam Carey's view is that giving women a standardised supplement is a bit like giving all of us a size 5 pair of shoes. For some they may fit very well, for others they are hopeless. He's concerned that we may be wasting a lot of money on supplements which we may not need. We spend £280 million a year on vitamin and mineral supplements in the UK alone and that doesn't include mail order or health-food shop sources. Ironically, it's those who may most need supplements, the elderly and the poor, both of whom tend to have poor diets, who are least able to afford them.

Dr Carey recommends consulting an expert. At his Harley Street clinic it costs £85 at the time of writing for a consultation with a doctor and a nutritionist. It is certainly worth consulting an expert, because if supplements are not balanced in the correct way they can create potentially dangerous nutritional cocktails.

In *The Hormone Dilemma* Dr Susan Love advises, 'Do your research. A vitamin advertisement may claim to have "everything a woman needs", but that doesn't mean it's true. Once you find a combination that truly provides you with the appropriate supplements, stick to it, while you keep trying to improve the variety and healthfulness of your diet.'

MENUS FOR A MENOPAUSE DIET

Judith Wills is the author of *The Food Bible*, the most authoritative work available on dietary needs for different age groups. It's a comprehensive and attractive guide to food and nutrition. She proves that it is not necessary to eat a boring or dull 'brown' diet in order to get the maximum benefit from food, and has designed this typical week's menu to give an idea of how you might put together an enjoyable and varied diet for your well-being and the whole family's enjoyment, rich in nutrients and phyto-oestrogens.

For breakfast have muesli, Weetabix, shredded wheat or porridge (and coffee – oops, naughty – Judith says only decaf!). Substitute half your weekly intake of dairy milk with a soya product. Add an orange or pink grapefruit or other citrus fruit, a few chopped nuts, preferably Brazil nuts, a dessertspoon of sesame or sunflower seeds and a good dessertspoon of wheatgerm. If you're still hungry, have a slice of wholegrain bread with a little butter and honey or Marmite.

MONDAY

Lunch

Salad of mixed green leaves (some dark green, e.g. rocket, lamb's lettuce, watercress) with celery, cucumber, tomato, a hard-boiled egg and 2 anchovies. Dress in olive oil and vinegar. Serve with wholemeal, rye or white bread. Finish with a banana.

Evening meal

CHICKEN CACCIATORE

Heat a tablespoon of olive oil in a flameproof casserole or heavy frying pan with a lid and brown 4 skinned, part-boned chicken thighs on all sides. Turn the heat down a little and add a crushed garlic clove and a few sprigs of fresh thyme, tarragon and oregano and 100ml (3½ fl oz) dry white wine. Stir for a minute or two. Add a small can of chopped tomatoes with their liquid and some black pepper. Bring to the boil, reduce heat, simmer and cook, covered, for 20 minutes or until the chicken is tender. Add 6 stoned and halved black olives, and 6 rinsed and drained capers, and cook for a further 2 to 3 minutes, until you have a little thick sauce left. Adjust the seasoning, adding a little sea salt if necessary.

Brown rice

Brussels sprouts or spring greens

Fruit and soya yogurt

TUESDAY

Lunch

Salad of drained tuna in oil mixed with cooked butter beans, sliced ripe tomatoes, red onion and lightly cooked asparagus tips, garnished with olive oil, red wine vinegar and chopped parsley. Serve with French bread.

Evening meal

STIR-FRIED TOFU

SPINACH, BROCCOLI AND WALNUT STIR-FRY

Blanch 100g (4oz) broccoli broken into florets in boiling water for 1 minute. Drain and refresh in cold water. Dry on kitchen paper. Heat 10ml (2tsp) walnut oil in a small nonstick pan and stir-fry the broccoli for 2 minutes. Add 100g (4oz) baby spinach leaves, a tablespoon of chopped walnuts, a teaspoon of sea salt and black pepper and stir-fry for 1 minute. Add 30ml (2tbsp) of vegetable stock towards the end of cooking.

Brown rice

Berry fruits with yogurt

WEDNESDAY

Lunch

LENTIL AND SPRING GREEN SOUP

Heat a tablespoon of groundnut oil in a saucepan and sauté a finely chopped medium red onion, until soft. Add a finely chopped garlic clove and stir for 1 minute. Add 500ml of good quality vegetable stock, 100g (4oz) (dry weight) of dark brown or Puy lentils and a chopped medium carrot, and bring to the boil. Reduce heat and simmer and cook for 30 minutes or until lentils are tender. Add a teaspoon of sea salt and black pepper, stir in a serving of raw spring greens, or alternatively, 30ml (2tbsp) of chopped coriander, and cook lightly. Add a tablespoon of reduced-fat Greek-style yogurt. Serve with rye bread.

Dried apricots

Evening meal

Omelette

Pepper and onion salad

1 banana

Thursday

Lunch

SMOKED MACKEREL PÂTÉ WITH GREEN SALAD
RYE BREAD
Coleslaw made with white cabbage, carrot, onion, dried
apricots and mixed nuts dressed with low fat bio yogurt mixed
with lemon juice, a little honey and black pepper.

Evening meal

Pasta with broccoli and anchovies
Mixed salad with balsamic vinegar dressing
1 orange

Friday

Lunch

Hummus
Pitta Bread
Salad of cucumber, olives, tomatoes, onion and dark green
lettuce leaves

Evening meal

GRILLED SARDINES OR HERRING FILLETS
DRESSED WITH GINGER AND CORIANDER
Arrange 4 herring fillets on a plate and place in a Chinese
bamboo or conventional steamer. Sprinkle with 10ml
(2tsp) soy sauce, 2 tsp lemon juice, a teaspoon of freshly
grated root ginger, salt and pepper. Steam for a few minutes
over boiling water till cooked through. Serve with the
juices poured over and garnish with 10ml (2tsp) chopped
fresh coriander.

Peas
New potatoes
Fresh fruit of choice

SATURDAY

Lunch
Salad of slices of ripe avocado, tomato and halloumi cheese dressed with olive oil and red wine vinegar, seasoned and flashed under the grill for 1 minute.
Ciabatta bread
Selection of seeds and dried fruits, e.g. pine nuts, sunflower seeds, dried figs, dried peaches

Evening meal
Grilled salmon fillet coated with mixed herbs and grated root ginger
Brown rice
Mangetout peas
Green lentils with herbs

SUNDAY

Lunch
Feta cheese, stir-fried in sunflower oil to brown and served with black stoned olives and lemon juice
Salad of fresh beansprouts, carrot, celery, watercress, spinach and mixed chopped nuts in classic vinaigrette dressing
White bread

Evening meal

    Small amount of extra lean organic beef, cut into strips and stir-fried in sesame oil with a selection of mixed fresh vegetables, including chinese leaves, with ginger, garlic and soy sauce

    Egg thread noodles

    Fresh fruit salad with yogurt

You can drink unlimited quantities of water, freshly squeezed fruit and vegetable juices and have a couple of snacks every day between meals. These should consist of fresh nuts, seeds, fruit, dried fruit, fortified soya milk, low-salt rye crispbread with a little low-salt peanut butter or hummus.

EXERCISE

There is absolutely no debate about this. Exercise is good for you. *What Doctors Don't Tell You* says, 'Just about every menopausal symptom, plus osteoporosis, risk of stroke and risk of heart failure can be reduced through daily physical activity.'

It was something Jo Wagerman discovered quite late in life, but then it's never too late to begin. As a young overweight woman she was told by a Harley Street specialist not to exercise as it would make her hungry. She took the slimming pills he gave her and lost four stone, but looks back with horror on her gullibility. She reckons his advice did long-term damage to her metabolic rate. When she retired, at the age of 60, seven years ago, she determined that she would get fit. She suffers from arthritis and is at high risk of osteoporosis as both her mother and grandmother had it. She wasn't going to let herself seize or crack up.

Jo joined a gym and now does an hour five mornings a week. She swims 50 lengths whenever she can. She believes that the combination of HRT, good diet and exercise is what has kept her physically strong and energetic. She has lost weight, changed shape and looks wonderful. The HRT, she thinks, helps to boost her energy levels enough to enable her to do the exercise bike and the weightlifting and doing the exercise makes the HRT more effective, helping to stop any mental deterioration.

PHYSICAL AND PSYCHOLOGICAL BENEFITS OF EXERCISE

Hot flushes

Some small studies have shown that exercise can help to minimise hot flushes. In one example, 6 per cent of physically active women had hot flushes, compared with 25 per cent of women who didn't exercise regularly. Penny Heeley, whose exercise programme you can follow (p. 255), had fewer symptoms than anyone I've spoken to and she is unquestionably the fittest.

Insomnia, mild depression, fatigue, anxiety

Exercise can elevate the level of endorphins in the brain. These are the brain chemicals that help to improve mood and reduce anxiety.

Prolonged exposure to stress hormones can be damaging to health and means the adrenal glands are not working at their best. If the body has no physical outlet for inactive stress you can suffer from backache, shoulder pain, tension headaches, digestive problems, ulcers and high blood pressure.

Regular physical exercise also makes you physically tired. Dr David Ashton says it should be an integral part of any strategy for dealing with insomnia. Paradoxically, exercise can also help you to beat fatigue by giving you more energy and stamina. If, however, you don't feel energised by exercise and it makes your symptoms of exhaustion even worse, you may have a problem such as an underactive thyroid. If so, see a doctor.

Weight control

Together with healthy eating, exercise will help to burn off calories and regulate the appetite, and toning the muscles will keep you, literally, in better shape.

Muscles, joints and flexibility

When done properly, exercise improves strength, flexibility, mobility and suppleness. Moderate physical exercise helps to maintain the health of joints, but don't overdo it. We all know the ballet dancers, athletes and professional footballers who suffer from osteoarthritis because of the intense physical strain of over-training. Take care to warm up before exercise in order to avoid any strain and only exercise within your capabilities.

Diabetes

Exercise in general boosts the immune system, the lymphatic system and the ability of the body to keep blood sugar levels in balance – reducing the risk of developing Type 2 diabetes which tends to appear over the age of 40.

Breast cancer

Some evidence suggests that exercise can lower risk. It helps to keep body fat under control and may also offer protection before the menopause, because it lengthens the menstrual cycle, thus decreasing the overall amount of oestrogen the body is exposed to. It's also been suggested that physically active women have less ovarian, uterine and colon cancer than sedentary women.

Heart disease

The heart expert Dr David Ashton says women who are physically active have about a 50 per cent reduction in coronary heart disease, compared with women who are physically inactive.

Exercise lowers blood pressure and increases good cholesterol,

HDL. The rise is quite small, but has a large impact on the risk of heart attack. It also diminishes the tendency for blood to clot by reducing the production of a substance called fibrinogen and blood platelet stickiness. If you already have heart disease, exercise is still important, providing the form and intensity is appropriate and carefully monitored.

Good aerobic activities for the heart include brisk walking, jogging, swimming, racquet sports, aerobic workouts, hill walking, dancing, netball, etc. Yoga, golf, bowling and housework are not so good at protecting the heart, but are very good for balance and flexibility.

Osteoporosis

Women who exercise throughout their lives have stronger bones than their sedentary counterparts, but it's never too late to start exercising for bone density. The benefits come from regular repeated exercise. Weight-bearing exercise is especially good for bones – in other words, any activity where you are supporting the weight of your own body, e.g. brisk walking, walking upstairs, dancing, such as tap which requires some impact, jogging, aerobics, racquet sports, carrying shopping, gardening. Swimming and cycling are not weight-bearing. Be careful, post-menopausally, of high-impact skipping and jumping as it can be dangerous for the joints, knees, ankles and back.

Strength training with weights is good for empowering muscles and in turn is helpful to the bones. Miriam Nelson published research in 1994 which showed that strength training twice a week cuts the rate of fractures for post-menopausal women. It's best learned and practised in the gym with a qualified instructor. (Go on, there'll be lots of other gravity challenged companions there – not everyone is slim, lithe and 21, honest! And actually, the male ones are worth going for – feast your eyes!)

Balance training won't increase bone density, but can help to protect bone by improving co-ordination and preventing falls.

Finally, stretching is important to any well-rounded exercise programme in warming up and cooling down.

GETTING STARTED

If you haven't exercised for a while:

- Don't rush into it – build up gradually and aim for steady improvement.
- If you have any medical conditions such as back or knee pain, angina, high or low blood pressure or heart problems, consult a doctor first.
- Listen to your body – if it hurts, stop (feeling the burn is very Jane Fonda, very 1980s, very out of date). If you feel dizzy or have discomfort in the chest, stop.
- Don't exercise if you are ill.
- Warm up and down with simple stretches.
- Wear correct shoes and comfy clothing.

If you have heart disease or osteoporosis, talk to your doctor and ask for advice about exercise. Take care too of isometric exercise such as lifting heavy objects, shovelling snow and digging the garden. Dr David Ashton advises against it, as it can strain the heart. Begin instead with walking and then move on to swimming or cycling.

HOW MUCH EXERCISE AND WHAT KIND?

What you do will depend on your priorities. If, for instance, your concern is heart disease and osteoporosis, you will need to combine aerobic and weight-bearing exercise. You can combine the two with aerobics classes and the gym or brisk walking and intermittent jogging. If you cycle and swim, which are good for the heart, don't forget weight-bearing exercise too.

Dr David Ashton advises starting with brisk walking. He says, 'Evidence suggests that a brisk walk every day may offer health benefits normally associated with more vigorous exercise. One recent study found that a woman who walks briskly (3–4 miles per hour) for at least three hours a week can reduce her risk of heart attack and stroke by 454 per cent. All in all, brisk walking is great exercise and one that is available to almost everyone.' He recommends 30 minutes on preferably all days of the week, which can be split into chunks, e.g. 15 minutes' walk morning and evening (get a dog!).

Do build up slowly to moderate intensity. You can establish this with the 'talk test'. If you can hold a conversation, but feel a bit breathless, it's just right. If you can chatter easily, speed up, if you can't talk at all, slow down.

A more specific measurement is heart rate. A safe level for aerobic exercise is to work at around 70 per cent of your maximum heart rate. To work it out, subtract your age in years from 220, which will give you your maximum heart rate in beats per minute for aerobic sessions. You can measure your heart rate by taking your pulse at the wrist. To begin, work at 50 per cent of maximum.

TOO MUCH EXERCISE

Do be wary of over-exercising. At the menopause we need some extra body fat as a source of oestrogen. If you exercise too much you can put the body under more stress than the exercise is relieving. More nutritional demands will be made by the body and excessive exercise can cause sweating which results in the loss of important minerals. Balance and moderation in all things.

RELAXATION

This is very important for reducing stress. Breathing exercises can help with hot flushes. Yoga and meditation can be relaxing and yoga will keep you supple.

PENNY HEELEY'S EXERCISE PLAN

Penny Heeley is a qualified teacher who was hired in her forties (she's now in her fifties) by Ragdale Hall Health Hydro to teach classes. Rather cleverly, they recognised that a middle-aged woman would be a fantastic draw for the majority of their clientele who are also middle-aged women.

Penny devised this programme specially for this book. You can, of course, extend the length of time for the cardiovascular exercises, but I asked her for a 10-minute daily programme which most of us can fit into busy lives.

10-MINUTE BONE BUILDER

This sequence of stretching exercises should be performed at least five times a week.

Chest stretch
Sit or stand and place your palms at the top of your buttocks. Squeeze your shoulder blades together and feel the top of the chest opening out and stretching. This helps to prevent slouching.

Back stretch
Sit or stand and place lightly clasped hands in front of your shoulders away from your body and at shoulder height. Imagine that you are pressing your hands into a wall, but keeping your elbows ever so slightly bent. You should feel a stretch in your upper back between the shoulders.

Shoulder stretch
Sit or stand and place your right hand on your left shoulder with your right elbow at shoulder height. Place your left hand on your right elbow and gently pull on the elbow so that the

right hand moves over the left shoulder. You should feel a stretch across the shoulder. Repeat on the other side.

Abdominal stretch

Sit or stand. Pull your navel in towards your spine and place lightly clasped hands above your head. Push upwards, keeping your elbows slightly bent. You should feel a stretch coming from your abdomen, right up through the front of your torso.

Buttock and leg stretch

Stand on your left leg and place your right heel slightly forward, and the toes up. Bend your left knee, keeping the right leg straight. Press your bottom slightly backwards and down. You should feel a stretch all the way down the back of the leg. Repeat on the other side.

Quad stretch

Stand on one leg and bring the other heel back and up towards the buttocks. Squeeze your buttocks together and you should feel the stretch along the front of the thigh.

Note: Each stretch should be performed twice and held for 30 seconds without bouncing.

RESISTANCE EXERCISES

These exercises should be performed five times a week for maximum benefit.

Chest press (works chest, shoulders, arms, upper back)

Kneel on the floor with a folded towel beneath your knees. Your knees should be hip-width apart and directly under the hips. Place your hands on the floor, on a line with your shoulders, but slightly wider than shoulder-width apart. Pull in your abdominal muscles towards your spine and, slowly, with control, bend your elbows so that your nose almost touches the floor . . . then slowly return to the original position.

ALTERNATIVE for those with knee problems. This exercise can be performed standing against a wall. With your arms slightly wider than shoulder-width apart and raised at shoulder height, keep your feet in line with your hips, place your hands on a wall and bend your elbows until your nose almost touches the wall – then push away.

Twisting bicep curl (works forearms, biceps)

With a 2kg dumb-bell in each hand, stand with your feet hip-width apart, and your knees slightly bent. Pull your abdominal muscles in slightly to support your lower back. Place your arms by your sides with a slight bend at the elbow and your palms facing towards your thighs. Keep your elbows tucked into the side of the waist. With control, bring your dumb-bells up to shoulder height, twisting your hands so that the palms face upwards. Then lower the dumb-bells with palms upwards and halfway down, turn the palms downwards.

Lateral raise (works tops of shoulders and upper back)

Stand as for the twisting bicep curl. With the palms of your hands facing inwards and slightly bent at the elbows, raise your arms out to the side to shoulder height and then lower, with control.

Upright row (works upper back, arms and shoulders)

Stand as for the twisting bicep curl. Place your hands in front of your thighs with palms facing you. Raise your elbows as high as you can, past the ears if possible, keeping the dumb-bells lower than your chin . . . and lower with control. Keep stomach muscles tight . . . do not allow your bottom to stick out.

Abdominal squeeze

Stand with good posture and knees slightly bent and imagine you have a red dot painted 75cm (3in) below your belly button. Squeeze the dot in towards your spine without tightening your bottom, keeping good posture all the time. Do this as slowly as possible and keep the lower abdominals working.

Do 12 to 15 repetitions of these exercises. Remember to pull your abdominals into the spine to support the lower back. If you don't have dumb-bells you could use a 454g tin of baked bins, although the benefits will not be as good.

WEIGHT-BEARING AND CARDIOVASCULAR EXERCISES

Jumping

(Primarily for pre-menopausal women. Not for those with back, knee or ankle problems.)

Stand on the floor, feet hip-width apart. Bend both knees and jump in the air so that your feet are 75cm (3in) to 100cm (4in) from the floor. Land on the balls of your feet, allowing your heels to come into contact with the floor on landing. Bend your knees. To make it a little harder on jumping, raise your arms to shoulder level to give extra lift and lower them as you come down. Aim for 25 jumps to begin with and progress to 100.

OR

Brisk walking

Walk as briskly as you can for 5 minutes without stopping. You should feel a little out of breath when you stop.

OR

Stepping

Walk up and down the stairs for 5 minutes without stopping. Again, you should feel a little out of breath when you stop.

PENNY'S CHAIROBIC WORKOUT

This is designed for women who are recovering from illness, are very overweight, unused to exercise, 65 plus, or simply looking for a different type of exercise.

Checklist

Before beginning, ensure that:

- You are wearing loose clothing.
- The chair is a dining chair or stool without arms and your feet can comfortably touch the floor. If not, arrange a block, step or books on which to place your feet.
- The angle behind the knees should be 90 degrees.
- The room is warm.
- You have a glass of water to sip.
- If you play music, it isn't too fast.

The number of repetitions for each exercise is indicated in brackets. All should be performed in a controlled manner with no jerking movements. An asterisk* indicates that a 500g (1lb) handweight or tin of beans can be held in each hand.

For each exercise, sit well back in the chair with the backs of your thighs supported. Lengthen your spine, sit tall, relax your shoulders and allow your arms to hang by your sides. If you have to strain, you are trying too hard.

The warm-up

1. Flick fingers and hands downwards, then in front at shoulder height, then overhead, then in front, then down (8 flicks in each position). Tap toes and heels at the same time. (x 2)

2. Swing your arms forwards and upwards in a large arc. (x 4)

3. Roll your shoulders forwards (x 4). Roll them backwards. (x 4)

4. Turn your head to look right, then front, then left, then front. (x 4)

Repeat each one twice more.

Upper body workout

1. *Overhead press** Place your hands at ear level, then raise them towards the ceiling and lower them to ear level. (x 12)

2. *Bicep curls** Keeping your elbows into the sides of your body with your hands hanging down and made into a fist, thumbs turned outwards, raise your hands to shoulder level and back to the starting position. (x 12)

3. *Chest Press** Place your hands in front of your shoulders and push forwards until you feel a stretch in the upper back then return your hands to the starting position. (x 12)

4. *Tricep scissors** With the palms of your hands facing backwards, squeeze your shoulder blades together and press your hands up behind you. Keeping your arms up and behind you, scissor your hands behind your back. (x 12)

5. *Lateral raise** Allow your arms to relax downwards, by your sides, and with a slight bend in the elbow, bring your arms outwards and upwards to shoulder level then lower to the starting position. (x 12)

6. *Shoulder rolls** Roll your shoulders forwards, then backwards in as big a movement as you can. (x 12)

Mid-section workout

Check your sitting position while doing these!

1. *Side bends** Keep both buttocks in contact with your chair seat. Bend directly to one side to a count of 4, hold in place for 4 and then come up for 4. Repeat on the other side. (x 3)

2. *Baby rocking* Loosely grip your forearms with your hands, raise alternating elbows high from side to side as if rocking a baby. (x 12)

3. *Side twists* Keep your buttocks in contact with your chair seat. Place your hands in front of your shoulders and raise your elbows to shoulder height if possible. Keep your elbows high and gently twist to the left, then front, then right, then front. You may place your hands on your hips if you find this more comfortable. (x 12)

4. *Pelvic tilt* Sit tall. Press back gently into the back of your chair. Pull your tummy button towards the chair back and lift your pelvis slightly forward and upwards. This is a tiny movement. (x 12)

5. *Arm circles* Circle your arms forwards and backwards, one at a time, then both together. (x 6)

Lower body workout

Check your sitting position and repeat all exercises 12 times.

1. *Buttock squeeze* Sit tall, with your feet flat on the floor. Squeeze your buttocks tightly and then release.

2. *Knee lift* Lift and lower one knee, without allowing your foot to touch the floor until all repetitions are completed. Repeat on the other side.

3. *Leg extension* Raise one foot 2.5cm (1in) from the floor. Bring your lower leg up until your foot is aligned with your thigh and lower without your foot touching the floor until all repetitions are completed.

4. *Flex and point* Raise one foot 2.5cm (1in) from the floor. Flex your foot and point the toe. Repeat on the other side.

5. *PC Plod* Place your feet flat on the floor, with your feet and knees together. Open your toes whilst keeping your heels together – your knees will part at the same time. Bring your knees together.

6. *Pigeon toes* Place your feet flat on the floor, feet and knees together. Part heels, keeping your toes together. Bring your heels together.

7. *Toe taps* Keeping your heels on floor, tap the toes on your right foot and then repeat on the left foot.

8. *Heel raises* Raise your heels, keeping the balls of your feet on the floor, then lower.

9. *Ankle circles* Raise one foot from the floor and circle the toes clockwise, then anti-clockwise. Repeat on the other side.

ENJOY!

Chapter 8

Old age ain't for cissies

MENOPAUSE

Now and again –
Since I was quite young –
I reckon my quota of seed
That we stopped from growing: not, of course,
All would have made it – there wasn't time
Nor strength in myself. But I think of them.

We raised three – and couldn't really have done
With more. It just feels strange
I might have had a dozen
Persons in my gift: and who would they have been?

In school biology, we were told once
How the female seeds are laid down at her making:
   one to go
Every month, when her body's ready,
Taking its chance.

I remember sniggers – also, myself
Looking from the window
Even as I smirked. What a day it was,
Blue and white . . .
And the thing seemed wonderful.
Seed by seed, lined up for years,
Waiting in the dark for the blind push
To be someone. More curious to me
Than the well-known puzzles,
Everyone's go. God – the stars . . .

I don't suppose Jack ever gave a thought
To such ideas. Men are so wasteful,
Careless of their seed. I often guess
What lives those might have had
Given some luck.

The colours of their eyes . . .

Jean Earle (b. 1909)

I first read this wonderful poem in 1996 when it appeared in a collection compiled by an old friend, Pat McGloughlin, for the BBC *Woman's Hour* 50th Anniversary Poetry Collection. I was 46 and beginning to have the first inklings of my own impending menopause. It made me cry and I sobbed out my own regret for my 'quota of seed', now coming to its natural end. I had not even realised, before I read the poem, that there would be sadness at the passing of my fertility. I have raised two and couldn't really have done with more either, but it is the shock of this grief, more than any of the other physical changes of the menopause, which, I now believe, affects us all profoundly, whether we are mothers or not.

Joan Bakewell confesses that she harboured a germ of panic when she realised she was crossing a Rubicon from which there was no return. Her children were grown up and she 'sort of minded' there would never be another pregnancy. It was a rite of passage and inevitable, but it took a while to accept that her sense of herself as a feminine woman was undiminished. In the end she decided she could worry about it and become depressed if she wanted, but she didn't want to. So she gave herself a good talking to, comforted herself with the pleasure of not having periods and enjoying an energetic sex life without worrying about contraception and carried on regardless.

Eve Pollard, whose children are now also grown up, tells me she too suffered pangs that there would be no more babies, even though it was the last thing she wanted. She also described the absence of something her friend, the journalist Anne Leslie, calls the 'white noise' which used to occur at parties. It is, she says, 'That buzz of interest when blokes look at you. It stops!' When she became depressed for a time, she realised it was not without a reason and that she needed to redefine herself.

Janet Balaskas who, as founder of the Active Birth Movement, is constantly surrounded by reminders of fecundity, became quickly aware that her menopause was an important spiritual journey, just as her adolescence and four pregnancies had been. For her, it was a surprisingly long transition, five years, where she came to terms with her own declining fertility, getting older, the death of people close to her and her own mortality. It was only by facing the tough realities and putting a great deal of thought into managing the physical changes her menopause brought that she began to feel she was far from old, but had passed over a significant hurdle. She was stronger, wiser and empowered to put her wisdom to good use. It's apparent from all my conversations with friends and with the contributors to this book that we need to give ourselves time to grieve for the women we were and acquaint ourselves with the potential of the women we have become.

There is much talk now of reversing or delaying the menopause, although newspaper stories which claimed it was possible to peform an ovarian graft, citing the case of Margaret Lloyd White, a 30-year-old infertile dancer, were found to have been premature. The graft did not restore her fertility. Nevertheless, as technology advances at an unimagined pace, there is no doubt it will come and sooner than we think. In Massachusetts, USA, reseachers have successfully removed from mice a gene which is connected to cell death and some of their eggs remained viable enough to be fertilised *in vitro*. There is the potential to delay the menopause in women by chemical means. The drug company Organon in Holland is working on a pill that will block the production of FSH, the follicle stimulating hormone. Its purpose is to act as a contraceptive, but it may, in the long term, put off the menopause by slowing down the process of egg loss.

These moves have been welcomed by the British Pregnancy Advisory Service who say women in their fifties and sixties may well be embarking on a second or third marriage and may want to reproduce with a new partner. Personally, I can't think of anything worse than saddling a child with a parent who should be looking forward to the gentler and slightly more distanced relationship of grandparent (of either sex, it has to be said. I'm no supporter of the Charlie Chaplin or Michael Douglas school either). I'm with the 1990 Human Fertilisation and Embryology Act which says the welfare of a possible child should be paramount.

It seems to me a supremely selfish act to have a child for whom you are unlikely to be able to do your best. The fittest 60-year-old can't conceivably be up to night-time feeds, nappies and playing football in the park – followed by a 20-year commitment to developing another personality. It's hard enough coping with teenagers in your forties and fifties. Dealing with mood swings, running a taxi service and grappling with the anxiety of the generation gap is exhausting. A two- or three-generation gap can be good for neither party. Research carried out in doctors' surgeries suggests mine is the majority view. Most female patients say they have learned to revel in a fit and healthy middle and old age without the fear of pregnancy.

Not that there's anything wrong with selfishness for its own sake. As long as no one else gets hurt by it, now seems the perfect time to 'do your own thing'. It might be getting a job after staying at home for years, packing up the job and taking to the open road, easing into the pleasure of being a grandparent, becoming a school governor or a local councillor, or taking on an even bigger job than the one you have. If there are no elderly parents to be cared for and the children have flown the nest, the possibilities are endless.

In this sense, we are truly the beneficiaries of almost a century and a half of our predecessors who have given us a template for taking our place in public life and using our experience as older women. They're women like James Miranda Barry, who was the first British female to qualify as a doctor. She had to dress as a man to study in Edinburgh and spent her entire career as an army physician by fooling the authorities into thinking she was male. Her true sex was only discovered on her death in 1865. She was 70. In the same year, Elizabeth Garrett Anderson, the first British woman to qualify as a doctor in her own guise, completed her training in France. She was elected dean of the London Medical School for Women in London when she was 47 and was active in medicine and the suffragette cause until her death at 81 in 1917.

At the time of writing there are numerous prominent women leading where we might follow. There's Barbara Castle, fighting vociferously for pensioners' rights in the year of her 90th birthday, her forensic debating skills undiminished. Teresa Gorman came into politics in her fifties by knocking ten years off her age to avoid any ageism among her selection committee. At 67, she's planning to stand down from her seat at the next election, because she's fed-up with being stuck on the back benches and wants to give herself an opportunity to do 'some other career', as yet unspecified. There is, she says, no question of running out of steam or getting ready to join the club of the retired.

Jo Wagerman, at 67, became the first woman to be elected president of the Board of Jewish Deputies in the summer of 2000. She has blossomed in her late middle age. She's fitter and more visible than at any other time in her life and tells me she gets outrageous compliments on her looks and her smartness, especially in Europe! Janet Paraskeva, at 54, and with a lifetime of big jobs behind her, latterly running the National Lottery Charities Board, began to think of slowing down. The idea of maybe working three days a week and increasing her time on the golf course was looking quite attractive when she was headhunted for the new post of chief executive at the Law Society. She was described in a newspaper article as the kind of woman who when shown 'a poisoned chalice would probably swig it in one go, but only after checking quietly the antidote she took earlier was the correct one.' All thoughts of semi-retirement were put aside. 'I realised,' she told me, 'the process of ageing is serious stuff, but I wasn't ready to slow down yet. There was time for one more big challenge.'

Shirley Williams is 70 years old and running a transatlantic life as an active Liberal Democrat peer in Britain and a professor of Politics at Harvard University. She began living in Britain and America when she married Professor Richard E. Neustadt of Harvard in 1987. When I asked her how she had coped with her busy life through middle age and beyond she said, 'Getting older in public life is so secondary. If you see yourself only as a sexual, reproductive being, I'm sure it's very hard when that part is behind you. But for me, even as a mother, it was only one part – I've always been valued, and valued myself, for other things.'

But I doubt there are many of us who can accept our ageing selves as gracefully and as naturally as Shirley has. It's a shock every time I walk past a mirror or shop window and see echoes of my grandmother, who was my current age when I was a little girl and looked the way women in their fifties and sixties were then supposed to look. She was round, grey-haired and sported the hairstyle still worn by the Queen – curly and combed into two little horns on the forehead. It made her look 90 long before her time. She wore sensible shoes, staid frocks and pinnies. She was comforting, warm, loving and wholeheartedly devoted to her family. I adored her, but I don't want to look like her and I don't want my horizons defined by the walls of my kitchen.

So who do we want to be and what do we want to look like? We've already considered these questions in relation to HRT, as its reported effects on collagen in the skin and boost to energy levels may be a consideration in deciding whether or not to take it. Equally we need to choose whether we want to grow old as young as possible – dyeing our hair, lifting our faces, dieting and exercising ourselves into slender, muscular middle age and wearing mini skirts in our dotage – or be content to become plump and comforting, wearing our grey hair and wrinkles with pride. Or is mix and match an option?

I, for instance, am not too fussed about the thickening waistline and chubbier chops, but I invest a queen's ransom every six weeks in a superb hairdresser who cuts beautifully and employs the best colourist in London. She's lightened my naturally very dark hair a couple of tones and put in highlights. (If it's dyed too dark it looks terrible against ageing skin.) Teresa Gorman agrees that a good hardresser is vital. She says she's grey as a badger, but hasn't seen it for ages. She too has lighter colour hair because it's kind to wrinkles and admits to vain delight every time there's a gasp of amazement when she tells people her age.

I buy a few good clothes each year and dress them up with expensive and elegant scarves and pashminas. The novelist Maggie Grahame says she learned a great deal about how to dress as a *femme d'un certain âge* when she won a prize for her writing which paid for her to spend a sabbatical in France. It was in the local tabac that she noticed the owner, a woman of Maggie's age, dressed for work in trousers and shirt, looked elegant, chic and sexy. As Maggie had put on middle-aged spread, she'd gone shopping for clothes and a little voice in her head would whisper, 'There's nothing for you here, come on Maggie, you're a granny.' When she began to look her age she lost her confidence. When she looked for role models she found Germaine Greer wanted her to wait around to be a crone and the alternative was Tina Turner. As she didn't want either she 'wimped out and became invisible'. When her doctor offered her Prozac for menopausal symptoms of depression she told him she 'needed her misery' for her writing, declined and went home to weep.

So, she asked herself, why hadn't these middle-aged French-women given up? She befriended a couple, Françoise and Corinne, and says she will never forget Corinne, just back from work, shrugging out of her raincoat, kicking off her shoes and saying, 'Would a glass of champagne be OK?' Such style!

Under the tutelage of Françoise and Corinne, Maggie bought perfume and lingerie, had her hair restyled and coloured and had a manicure. She bought a soft leather bag and some silk scarves from a street market and found stylish clothes that fitted her fuller figure in a department store. The French, she observes, have no youth culture that tells women it's fine to grow older as long as you don't look it, dearie, so they feel comfortable dressing their age.

Joan Bakewell and Gloria Hunniford simply have a talent for choosing the right kind of clothes for their age. Gloria looks after her skin, on the advice of an air hostess friend, with Lancôme's Hydrix. It would, she says, shrivel without it. She would have a facelift, but isn't yet brave enough, so she's holding it in reserve. She never goes out without her make-up and has always been a classic, rather than a trendy dresser. She always wears shoulder pads to square off her rounded shoulders, buys cheap black skirts and spends all her money on jackets which she dresses up with scarves and brooches. Joan looks after her eyebrows, nails and legs. Her hair, she says, is floppy, a problem to be solved, not her crowning glory. She has a professional haircut and uses henna for colour. Whilst she wouldn't describe herself as narcissistic, she always tries to apply the basic principles of good grooming and, like Gloria, chooses classic clothes which look as attractive for 60 as they did for 50.

Big jewellery is also useful as you get older; anything that will continue to get you noticed, but distract attention from the bits you'd rather hide. Diamonds, especially, always look so common on the young and fabulously glamorous on older, perfectly manicured hands. And yes, you can afford a manicure, these days. There's not nearly so much washing up to do when the young have flown the nest, so it's not a waste of money. Have a pedicure too – looking after your feet is not an indulgence, but a necessity now – and it feels great to be pampered.

Eve Pollard's changing feet have been one of her biggest worries. For her daughter's wedding, she bought spectacularly high heels, the kind she wore every day when she was younger, to 'sashay in', but made sure she had a comfy pair of much lower ones for the evening. If your feet hurt, she says, you won't enjoy yourself. She's delighted to see kitten heels are back in fashion – as she flicked through *Vogue* and saw them on display she told herself 'I can do that!' She also indulged in Botox injections for the wedding, which, she says, were brilliant for stopping her frown lines. She's not worried about any possible toxic effect of having botulism injected into her face as it's now done so widely; she thinks it's safe, but she is hesitating over having it done again, as her face 'might go wonky'.

When I researched my last book – a history of women in Britain since the Second World War – I was surprised and encouraged at the results of a survey I carried out asking who were the women we wanted to look like. I expected most of us would say Marilyn Monroe, Isabella Rossellini, Ava Gardner, Joan Collins, Helen Mirren or Gloria Steinem – all significant beauties, and those who survived into middle age were as youthful looking in their fifties and sixties as in their thirties. Contrary to my assumptions, the two names which came up most frequently were Glenda Jackson and Judi Dench, admired, I was told, because they had allowed themselves to age naturally, but were elegant and wore their character in their faces. I'm sure, too, that the women of the Rylstone WI, whilst starting an unfortunate trend in less attractive nude calendars than theirs, have, nevertheless, contributed to our reclaiming the right to look lovely while looking our age.

Glenda, interestingly, is utterly without vanity, but she's also very lucky. She notices very little physical change in herself and so far, in her sixties, has only two grey hairs. She finds exercise repellent, working on the principle that if you can't stand sit, if you can't sit lie, but probably keeps fit doing her own housework. She has, she says, no strong sense of being sexually attractive and found the fact that the British press turned her into a sex symbol very funny. Her appearance has never much concerned her as it's always been in the hands of others who made of her whatever character they wanted. The real Glenda Jackson says she is just a hardworking politician who dresses neatly, gets her energy from honey and wheatgerm and simply gets on with what needs to be done.

She wouldn't consider a facelift. Angela Rippon agrees. Even though her business in television and radio (and mine) seems to require its men to be craggy and well worn, flaunting their age and experience, and its women fresh-faced and girlish (Teresa Gorman says it always infuriates her that at middle age men are considered to be in their prime and women over the hill), she wouldn't submit herself to the knife, partly out of terror. She broke her nose during her years of competitive riding and has had plastic surgery on it three times. It was such agony, there's no way she would go through it all again purely for vanity. But she does give herself whatever help she can.

Angela takes care with her diet and exercises regularly, a habit she developed as a young dancer. She accepts that she can't expect, at 56, to look the way she did at 36. She hasn't fallen into the trap of trying to look like the 'tele totties' and is proud of her crow's feet and laughter lines because she has earned them. Nevertheless, she says, it isn't cheating destiny to want to look good and take advantage of what's out there. Her greasy skin, she thinks, has helped to keep lines at bay, but she believes facial acupuncture helps to keep the muscles tight and she goes regularly for a massage which uses an electrical charge on the wrinkles. She's convinced that ten years from now there will be a different set of attitudes as more women move into the ranks of senior management and television producers recognise that women like her, Anna Ford, Anne Robinson and Julia Somerville have a great deal to offer. They turn up on time, are well-informed and can do the job. Other older women, moreover, like to see themselves reflected on the screen.

Vera Ivers from the Older Women's Network is angered by what she describes as the media's requirement that if they are going to show an older woman she must look like Joan Collins, or have climbed Everest or rowed across the Atlantic. Vera doesn't dye her hair, take HRT or battle with her wrinkles. She wasn't sure who she was trying to impress and, frankly, found it wasn't worth the hassle. She exercises three times a week at a women's gym, but that's to keep fit, not young. You can't, she told me, be a 20-year-old for the rest of your life.

Once she had got over the short period, during her menopause, when she felt less attractive and less sexy, she decided to make the most of who she had become, naturally. She began to find women of her own age good company and realised that for the first time in her life she wasn't concentrating all her energies on men. She would, she thought, be attractive in her own way. Then she began to notice other older people and enjoy the life's experience she could see in their faces. She found that when people have done and seen so much their faces respond much more interestingly in conversation than someone whose face is tightened by surgery.

As a local councillor, Vera became very aware of the dying of the 'white noise' of sexual chemistry which Eve Pollard mentioned and realised she had to find new strategies for getting what she wanted. She noticed younger women flirting and being courted by men and felt cross with them because they seemed to be demeaning themselves. But it was quickly apparent that the men she worked with didn't know any other roles for women than sex object or mother. So she played the maternal card and deliberately set out to 'collect young men' who might be useful to her. She listened to their troubles and invariably got her own way. After all, she laughs, they're not going to argue with their mother, are they?

Like Vera, Janet Paraskeva has found she likes the way older women look (and I have to say, of all the women I have interviewed in the past few months, two stand out in my mind – the philosopher, Baroness Warnock, and the birth guru, Sheila Kitzinger. Both are in their seventies. Their hair is grey and a little wild. They are wrinkled, but their faces shine out with humour, energy and the confidence that comes with experience). Janet likes her own grey hair and her wrinkles don't bother her. She used to have pink streaks, but she's abandoned those and says she's never flirted to get on. It's no way to manage. Her straightforward approach has brought her the respect and support of women colleagues which she finds invaluable. She dresses smartly for the office, in a Nicole Farhi suit, because appearance matters – it's what people see – but it doesn't inspire confidence in a high-powered job if it says inexperienced girl or glamour puss.

How, though, do we manage our relationships with the men at home? The stories of women who are left by their husbands or partners at around this time are legion. It's my conviction that middle-aged men practise a form of cannibalism when they trade in the old model for a new and shiny one, believing they can gobble up all that youth and beauty and rejuvenate themselves. Regrettably, there are enough young women out there who fall into their trap of power and wealth and end up as nursemaids, but that's not our story. There's comfort, though, in the knowledge that one day ours will be theirs.

Some women find it hard to recover from the grief and humiliation of being left alone. Sandy Chalmers says she still grieves for her loss and has avoided relationships since she and her husband separated because she couldn't bear to be hurt like that again. She busied herself instead with her job as director of communication at Help the Aged and her charity work with the Pennell Initiative for Women's Health. She thinks financial independence and being able to afford to buy her husband's share of their home was a great comfort. She also found she was able to rediscover a friendship with her ex when she helped out when her mother-in-law was ill. Family ties are stronger than we think. She and her sister Judy shared the care of their mother, although she hardly needed it. 'Milly', says Sandy, 'lived till the day she died. She didn't think she could get a job when our father died when she was in her early forties, but she did and it knocked years off her age. She should have retired years before she did, but she just put on more eye shadow.' An example her daughter intends to follow.

Vera Ivers is impatient with men who run off to pastures new. It happened to her, but she reflects, philosophically, that it doesn't say much for the relationship if he leaves you. She found someone else to share her life – a man 12 years her junior. He kept her young for a while, but then seemed to catch up in his fifties and she found to her relief that her mum and aunts distorted the truth when they claimed sex came to an end post-menopause. She went off it a bit during her menopause, but then regained her interest. 'There have been some changes,' she giggles, 'he can't keep it up all night and we rest for a few days in between, but mostly it's comforting and comfortable.' (I was delighted to read recently that the actress Shirley MacLaine, when asked at a party whether she still has sex in her sixties, threw her glass of wine over the impertinent young man and replied, 'Yes, but not with someone as wet as you!')

The novelist Rosie Thomas is one of those amazing women who do climb mountains after their menopause. She found she had a wonderful feeling of freedom once she had 'done the mothering bit'. She did the Peking to Paris car rally and plans to climb Everest soon 'even if I have to do it on a Zimmer frame'. But it was after the car rally that her husband of 30 years left her, suddenly and without warning. Like Sandy Chalmers, she grieved for their shared history and says it was the little things that really got to her: having to replace dead light bulbs, decide which estate agent to use or work out whether or not she could afford a new car. She has discovered, though, it's easier to be selfish on her own and pursue her travel and climbing interests. She has a new boyfriend, which reassured her that she was still attractive and the sex is fine. She's not asking whether or not it will last, but finds it's good to have someone with whom she can go to the theatre. She remains friends with her husband and says she has learned a new philosophy. After 25 years of always looking forward, mostly on behalf of her children, she now finds it's OK to live in the present.

Similarly, Edwina Currie, whose marriage broke up when she famously said her husband liked to stay at home in the evenings and watch TV whilst she preferred to be on it, has found herself a new man. John is a police officer whom she met through her radio programme on Radio 5 Live. He was in a studio in the Midlands and she was in London. She fell in love with his voice and now finds herself blooming because she is loved and in love. Her advice to anyone who is in a loveless relationship is to be brave and get out. HRT, she thinks, won't get the juices going, but there may be someone out there who will.

Gloria Hunniford found her new romance, after some years of being alone, when she was 58. She had had other relationships, but they never seemed right and she never wanted to marry again. But she did when she met Steven. At first they were good friends and for about a year simply liked each other. She describes it as an old-fashioned teenage courtship, but the love, when they acknowledged it, was different. It was comfortable, fulfilling, sweet and considerate of each other's needs and feelings. As far as sex after 60 goes, it's a fallacy, she tells me, that we go off it. Her husband had a heart attack last year, which can be a worry, but it's manageable.

Some of the women I've spoken to are, like me, lucky to have a long-term relationship with a man with whom they hope to grow old. Eve Pollard has been married for 21 years and says it gives her great confidence to be with a man who fancies and loves her. She can't imagine how dreadful it would be to be going on the pull, but is reassured that her husband seems to like her for what's in her brain as much as for the externals. She looks forward to them ageing together, worrying about getting enough exercise and eating the right foods as a pair and to laughing with the man who knew her when she was young and energetic.

Some of the women have contented partnerships with other women. Angela Mason and Janet Paraskeva both spoke of the comfort of sharing your ageing with someone of your own sex who really understood the physical changes. It can still be tough to deal with other people's attitudes to lesbian relationships and in Angela's case, as she and Elizabeth have a teenage daughter, there are continuing worries about childcare – there can be no assumption that the 'woman' will stay at home – and supporting

her financially through school and university past the normal age
of retirement. Angela feels the three of them have a more open,
closer and more intimate relationship than many of the
heterosexual families she observes and of all the women I've
spoken to who have to deal with teenage children during their
middle years, theirs seems to be one of the most harmonious
households.

Angela Rippon is a contented singleton, full of juicy little titbits
of advice. She recommends an elegant fan for coping with hot
flushes, a tip she was given by Katie Boyle. When Angela asked her
whether she had ever taken HRT she said, 'No, darling, I never
take anything. Fans, darling, fans.' Angela describes it as a
wonderfully feminine reaction (jolly good idea too. I've tried it, in
a very hot theatre, and it's much more elegant than flapping a
programme!) Angela has been alone for 13 years since the
amicable separation from her husband, Chris. She now keeps her
private life private as Chris hated the publicity that went with
being Mr Angela Rippon and she's determined not to inflict it on
anyone else, but for the moment she's content to be alone. She has
lots of friends who are widowed, and others, both male and female,
who are single. She is self-sufficient, has saved and planned her
finances well to ensure a comfortable old age and often discusses
with her friends how they will support each other into old age. Her
godson (she has no children of her own) promises to take care of
her, but she doesn't want to be in a position where she has to be
looked after. She will, she says, deal with that one when it comes.

There are, of course, some men who are prepared to confess that
it's tough for them to get older too. Alan Clark in his diaries
bemoans his wrinkly face and says no girl ever gives him a passing
glance any more. The actor Charles Dance, once known as the
British Robert Redford, told me that he had felt 'menopausal'
when he turned 50. He wasn't sure whether it was hormonal or
simply that sense of being 50 and wondering, Oh, my God, now

what, but he felt dreadfully anxious and tired for a year or so. He, like so many women, was worried that he had been defined for so long through his looks and wondered what would happen as they began to fade. He is determined not to submit his face to the surgeon's knife and happily takes on parts where he is required to play men much older than himself.

There's been much talk in the press recently of the male menopause – a misnomer, of course, since men cannot have an end to their menstrual cycle as they don't have one – but research does suggest that there are hormonal changes in men and male hormone replacement therapy is being taken increasingly seriously. I am prepared to accept that they have a tough time too and deserve a little sympathy. I'm trying hard not to gloat and say, Hey, welcome to the club of tough decisions.

I have found writing this book infuriating at times as it is apparent that an awful lot of women are not getting an open-minded and sympathetic hearing or the best and most up-to-date advice about the range of options available to them when they arrive at the first port of call, the GP's surgery. The provision of specialist menopause clinics is woefully inadequate and good, long-term research on HRT and the alternatives is long overdue. On the other hand, talking to the women who have been so generous with their time and their stories about themselves and their personal circumstances has been a comfort and an inspiration. I've noticed, too, little glimmers of a more open attitude to the condition that until now dared not speak its name. I cheered when Julie Walters, interviewed on *Parkinson*, described bursting into tears when she was filming the dance sequence for the film *Billy Elliott* because she was menopausal. When I asked her about discussing her menopause on prime-time TV she howled, 'Jenni, I talk about my menopause all the time.' Good for her. The playwright Kay Mellor managed to bring it into her prime-time series drama *Fat Friends*, in which the women would meet in the loo of their slimming club and discuss whether or not to take HRT. One character memorably delivered this line: 'My mother used to call it the change – you change from a normal human being to a rottweiler!' And why not?

You may be wondering how I chose the title of this chapter. It was that interview with Bette Davis again, back in the late 1980s, and only a few months before her eightieth birthday and her death. She had already had a couple of strokes and a heart attack (she still smoked, as I recall, the cigarette held between her perfectly manicured bright red fingernails). When I asked her about her age, her health and her still immaculately elegant appearance, she held me with those terrifying eyes and said, 'People expect it. I'm a star and I learned early on in my career that my fans want to see a star. So I make the effort, no matter how terrible I feel. But you know, old age ain't for cissies. It's tough.' It's time now to toughen up and get ready.

BIBLIOGRAPHY AND
FURTHER READING

The Healthy Heart Handbook for Women Ashton, Dr David (Vermilion, 2000)

Menopause and Culture Berger, Gabriella E. (Pluto Press, 1999)

Hysterectomy and the Alternatives Clark, Jan (Vermilion, 2000)

The Menopause Industry Coney, Sandra (The Women's Press, 1995)

No Change Cooper, Wendy (Arrow, 1996)

Aromatherapy: an A–Z Davis, Patricia (Daniel, 2000)

Natural Alternatives to HRT Glenville, Marilyn (Kyle Cathie, 1997)

Natural Alternatives to HRT Cookbook Glenville, Marilyn (Kyle Cathie, 2000)

The Change Greer, Germaine (Penguin, 1992)

The Menopause, HRT and You Hawkridge, Caroline (Penguin, 1999)

A Change for the Better Jones, Dr Hilary (Hodder & Stoughton, 2000)

Passage to Power Kenton, Leslie (Vermilion, 1998)

What Your Doctor May Not Tell You About Menopause Lee John R., MD (Warner Books, 1996)

The Hormone Dilemma Love, Dr Susan (Thorsons, 1997)

Is HRT Right For You? MacGregor, Dr Anne (Sheldon Press, 1993)

Eat to Beat Your Age Marshall, Janette (Hodder & Stoughton, 2000)

Strong Women, Strong Bones Nelson, Miriam E., PhD (Piatkus, 2000)

Menopause Without Medicine Ojeda, Linda (Thorsons, 1998)

The Breast Cancer Prevention and Recovery Diet Olivier, Suzannah (Michael Joseph, 1999)

Natural Progesterone Rushton, Anna and Bond, Dr Shirley A. (Thorsons, 1999)

The Silent Passage Sheehy, Gail (Harper Collins, 1993)

The Phyto Factor Stewart, Maryon (Vermilion, 2000)

Cruising Through the Menopause Stewart, Maryon (Vermilion, 2000)

Menopause Stoppard, Miriam (Dorling Kindersley, 1994)

Old Age in English History Thane, Pat (Oxford University Press, 2000)

Raging Hormones Vines, Gail (Virago, 1993)

Women and Health: Feminist Perspectives Wilkinson, Sue and Kitzinger, Celia (eds) (Taylor and Francis, 1994)

The Food Bible Wills, Judith (Quadrille, 1998)

Feminine Forever Wilson, Robert (Allen, 1966)

Understanding HRT and the Menopause Wilson, Dr Robert C. (Which? Books, 1999)

USEFUL ADDRESSES

Amarant Trust
Sycamore House, 5 Sycamore Street
London ECIY OSR
Helpline: 01293 413000 [Mon-
Friday 11 am-6pm]
*The Trust provides information and
advice about all aspects of the
menopause and HRT to women and
health professionals. The helpline is
staffed by trained nurses. The
Amarant Centre treats patients
referred to them by a GP or practice
nurse.*
Tel: 020 7401 3855

**Aromatherapy Organisations
Council**
PO Box 19834
London SE25 6WF
Tel: 020 8251 7912
www.aromatherapy-uk.org

Breast Cancer Care
Kiln House, 210 New Kings Road
London SW6 4NZ
Helpline: 0500 245 345
www.breastcancercare.org.uk

Breast Care Campaign
Blythe Hall, 100 Blythe Road
London WI4 OHB
Administration: 020 7371 1510

British Acupuncture Council
63 Jeddo Road
London W12 9HQ
Tel: 020 8735 0400
www.acupuncture.org.uk

**British Association of Nutritional
Therapists**
27 Old Gloucester Street
London WCIN 3XX
Tel: 01202 417121

British Heart Foundation
14 Fitzhardinge Street
London WIH 6DH
Tel: 020 7935 0185
www.bhf.org.uk

British Homeopathic Association
15 Clerkenwell Close,
London EC1R OAA
Tel: 020 7566 7800
www.trusthomeopathy.org

**British Medical Acupuncture
Society**
12 Marbury House, Higher Whitley
Warrington, Cheshire WA4 4QW
Tel: 01925 730727
www.medical-acupuncture.co.uk

British Nutrition Foundation
High Holborn House, 52-54 High
Holborn
London WCIV 6RQ
Tel: 0207 404 6504
www.nutrition.org.uk

Cancer BACUP
3 Bath Place, Rivington Street
London EC2A 3JR
Cancer information service: 020
7613 2121
Freephone cancer information service:
0808 800 1234
www.cancerbacup.org.uk

Carers National Association
20-25 Glasshouse Yard
London ECIA 4JS
Administration: 020 7490 8818
Carers Advice Line: Lo-Call 0345
573 369 (open l0am-12pm and
2pm-4pm Mon-Fri)
www.carersuk.demon.co.uk

**The Centre for Nutritional
Medicine**
114 Harley Street
London W1G 7JJ
Tel: 020 7224 5053
www.nutritionalmedicine.com
*Founded by Adam Carey. Offers
private consultations/NHS referrals
with a team of doctors, nutrionists and
dieticians. Specialises in women's
health, cardiovascular disease and
osteoporosis.*

Daisy Network
PO Box 392, High Wycombe
Buckinghamshire HP15 7SH
www.daisychain.org
*Premature menopause support and
information (please send a large SAE).*

Family Heart Association
7 North Road, Maidenhead
Berkshire SLY IPE
Helpline: 01628 628 638
[Tuesday-Friday 9am-3pm]
www.familyheart.org

Hysterectomy Association
Beech Mews, 51 Burton Road
Coton-in-the-Elms
Derbyshire, DE12 8HJ
Tel: 01283 763447
www.hysterectomy-
association.org.uk

Marilyn Glenville
The Natural Health Practice
Danegate, Bridge Green
Tunbridge Wells TN3 9JA
Tel: 01892 750511
www.marilynglenville.com

Menopause Clinic – Research Unit
Northwich Park Hospital
Watford Road
Harrow
Middlesex HA1 3UJ
Helpline: 020 8869 2877/3965

Miss Pitken's Menopause Clinic
Clementine Churchill Hospital
Sudbury Hill, Harrow
Tel: 020 8537 8430

National Endometriosis Society
50 Westminster Palace Gardens
Artillery Row
London SW1P 1RL
Helpline: 020 7222 2776
www.endo.org.uk

**National Institute of Medical
Herbalists**
56 Longbrook Street, Exeter
Devon EX4 6AH
Tel : 01392 426022
http://www.btinternd.com/-nimh

National Osteoporosis Society (NOS)
PO Box 10, Radstock
Bath BA3 3YB
Tel: 01761 471771 (for general enquiries)
Helpline: 01761 472721 (for medical queries)
www.nos.org.uk

Natural Progesterone Information Service
PO Box 24, Buxton
Derbyshire SKl7 9FB
Provides information packs on the use of natural progesterone and how to obtain it. Send a 1st class stamp for details.

Ovacome
St Bartholomew's Hospital
West Smithfield
London ECIA 7BE
Administration: 07071 781 861
www.ovacome.org.uk

Pennell Initiative for Women's Health
An organisation dedicated to promoting and co-ordinating research into older women's health.
Tel: 0800 550 220
www.pennellwomenshealth.org

Society of Homeopaths
4a Artizan Road
Northampton NNl 4AU
Tel: 01604 621400
www.homeopathy-soh.org

What Doctors Don't Tell You
4 Wallace Road
London Nl 2PG
Tel: 020 7354 4592
www.wddty.co.uk
Organisation that publishes a monthly newsletter taking a criticial look at conventional medicine and complementary alternatives.

Women's Health
52 Featherstone Street
London ECIY 8RT
Administration: 020 7251 6333
Health enquiry line: 020 7251 6580
(open 10.00am-4.00pm Mon, Wed, Thur, Fri)
An information centre for women's health issues, specialising in reproductive and sexual health.

Women's Health Concern
93-99 Upper Richmond Road
London SW15 2TG
Administration: 020 8780 3916
Helpline: 020 8780 3007
Helps women seek treatment and care for gynaecological conditions, in particular the menopause and hormone replacement therapy.

Women's Nutritional Advisory Service [WNAS]
PO Box 268, Lewes
East Sussex BN7 2QN
Tel: 01273 487 366
www.wnas.org.uk

INDEX

acupuncture 212
Agnus Castus 49
alcohol 88, 91, 229
Alendronate 93
Alzheimer's Disease 36, 147-9
angina 86
anorexia nervosa 26, 90
antioxidants 202, 231-3
anxiety 37, 250
aromatherapy 213-5
Australian women, menopausal symptoms 73

bioflavonoids 233
biphosphonates 93
black cohosh 207
black women, attitudes to menopause 67-8
bleeding problems 78-86
blood sugar level 221, 226
bones 31, 89, 90, 91, 149, 201, 234-40
bran, problems with 222, 236
breast cancer 72, 96-103, 162-8, 198-200, 251
breast lumps 34, 97, 98-103
breast screening 98-103, 165, 167
breasts, painful 34
BUPA, policy on hysterectomies 81

caffeine 33
calcitonin 94
calcium 234-6, 237-40
cancer 38-9 72, 78, 82, 96-103, 104-6, 162-8, 198-9, 230-4, 251
carbohydrates, complex 220-1
cardiovascular exercises 258-9
carotenoids 233
cervical cancer 104-6, 168
CHD (coronary heart disease) 38, 86-9, 152-8
cholesterol 38, 87, 154-5, 222, 223, 230
coffee 228
collagen loss 33
combined HRT, breast cancer risks 162-8

constipation 35
continuous combined HRT 120-21
contraceptive pill 22, 53, 116-7
coronary heart disease (CHD) 38, 86-9, 152-8
corticosteroids and osteoporosis risk 91
coumestans 193
Crinone 118, 127-8, 183
cystitis 95

decaffeinated coffee 228
dehydration 228
depression 21, 36, 37, 39, 146, 250
diabetes 26, 88, 251
diet 91, 216-49
diosgenin 183
doctors 61-3, 75-106
dong quai 208
drinks 229

ectopic pregnancy 79
embolisation 86
endometrial ablation 85
endometrial cancer 168, 187
endometrial hyperplasia 78
endometriosis 78, 82
equine oestrogen 114-6
ERT (estrogen replacement therapy) 53, 61 see also HRT
essential fatty acids (EFAs) 223-4, 238
Etidronate 93-4
evening primrose oil 206, 224
Evista (Raloxifene) 133-4
exercise 33, 88, 91, 250-62
eyesight and ageing 37-8

facial hair 29
fatigue 37, 250
fats 222-5
feminists 44, 55, 57, 62, 64-7, 70, 74
fibre 221-2
fibrocystic disease 34

fibroids 76, 82, 86
Filipino women, menopausal symptoms 73
fish oils 224, 231
flavonoids 232
FSH (follicle stimulating hormone) 10, 27, 28

genetically modified soya 196
gingko biloba 208-9
ginseng 209-10
glaucoma 38

hair 33, 144-5
Hazda women 69
HDL cholesterol 38, 87, 154, 223, 224, 230-1, 252
headaches 35
heart attack 87-8
heart disease 152-8, 202, 230-4, 251-2
heavy bleeding 78, 80-6, 179, 214
herbal medicine 205-6, 210
herbal teas 229
high blood pressure and CHD 88
homeopathy 212-3
hormone treatments, development of 52-5
hot flushes 23, 28, 31, 143, 228, 250
HRT (hormone replacement therapy) 30, 34, 38, 52-63, 72, 86, 88, 93, 94, 96, 108-41
    alternatives to 177-215
    pros and cons 142-76
human papilloma virus (HPV) 104
hypothalamus 26, 31
hysterectomy 23-4, 24-5, 80-6, 90
    alternatives to 85-6

incontinence 32-3, 94-6
insomnia 39, 250
intra-uterine device 79
iron 241
irregular bleeding, treatments for 80-6
irritable bowel syndrome 35
isoflavones 193, 201

Japanese diet 72, 192, 204, 219
joint pains 15

LDL cholesterol 38, 87, 154, 223, 224, 230-1
lesbian women, attitude to menopause 68-9
LH (luteinising hormone) 27, 28
life expectancy 44-6, 65
lignans 193
Livial (Tibolone) 132-3

magnesium 237
mammography 98-100
Mayan women, lack of menopausal symptoms 72-3
memory problems 15, 146-7
men, reactions to ageing 278-9
menopause 9,
    attitudes to 42-74, 263-6
    and diet 202-3, 242-9
    early 20-3, 90, 165-6
    late 26
menopause clinics 131, 140, 279
menorrhagia see heavy bleeding
menstrual cycle 26-7
microwave endometrial ablation 85
migraines 35
Million Women Study 80, 108, 156, 164-5, 167-8, 188
Mirena (inter-uterine system) 79-80, 129-31
miscarriage 79
mood swings, helped by HRT 146
muscle strength, and HRT 152
myomectomy 86

'natural' oestrogens 114
natural progesterone 178-90
natural therapies 177-215
needle biopsy 103
night sweats 14-16, 17, 28, 31, 143, 228

obesity 88, 225 see also weight
oestradiol 27, 112
oestriol 112
Oestrogel 126
oestrogen 26, 28, 30, 31, 32, 38, 62-3, 88, 90, 97, 112-16, 154, 157-8, 163, 178-9
oestrogen dominance 180-3, 184

oestrogen gel 127
oestrogen-only patch 122-5
oestrone 28, 112
older women 47, 267-78
Older Women's Network 46
omega 3 oils 224
omega 6 oils 224
oophorectomy 24
osteoporosis 30, 31, 72, 89-94, 133, 134,
    149-51, 200-1, 252
ovarian cancer 82, 168
ovarian cysts 79, 82
ovaries, sugical removal 14

pains 37
palpitations 14, 31
parenting later in life 266-7
Parkinson's Disease and oestrogen effects
    149
pelvic floor exercises 86, 94, 95
pelvic inflammatory disease (PID) 79, 82
perimenopause 14, 28, 36, 78-9, 138, 180
periods, stopped 9, 10, 11, 12
phytochemicals 232-3
phyto-oestrogens (POs) 72, 191-205, 227
placebo effect in treatment trials 169-70
polyps 79
potassium 238
pregnancy 9, 10
Premarin 114-6
Progest (natural progesterone) 183, 186
progesterone 32, 61, 117-8, 128, 178-90
progestogen 79, 117-8, 154, 159-60,
    167-8
prolapse of the uterus 82, 95
protein, sources of 225
psychological problems 35
Raloxifene (Evista) 133-4, 151
relaxation 254

sage 211
salt, in the diet 227
selenium 233-4
sequential combined HRT 119-20, 121

SERMs (selective oestrogen receptor
    modulators) 93, 133-4
sex 15, 16, 17, 18
skin 33, 144-5
smear test 104-5
smoking 22, 33, 88, 91
soya 193, 194-5, 201
St John's wort 210
stress 22-3, 35
sugar in the diet 226-7
supplements, views on 238-9, 242-4
surgery 24-5

tea 228-9
teeth and HRT 151
testosterone 28, 33, 34, 78, 134-5
Thai women, lack of menopausal
    symptoms 72
thyroid problems, symptoms 78
Tibolone (Livial) 132-3
transcervical resection of the
    endometrium (TCRE) 85

ultrasound scan, for breast screening 102,
    103
urinary problems 32-3, 94-6, 143-4

vaginal dryness 16, 18, 32, 143-4
venous thrombo-embolism risk, and HRT
    162
Viagra 59
vitamins 237-8, 240-1
voice, deepening of 29

water, drinking 230
weight 26, 34, 161-2, 251 see also obesity
wild yam 183, 184
women's movement 44 see also femininsts

xeno-oestrogens 180, 182

yoga 252, 254

zinc 242